Nursing

Nursing

Moving Forward

Douglas Long, RN, MBA, PhD

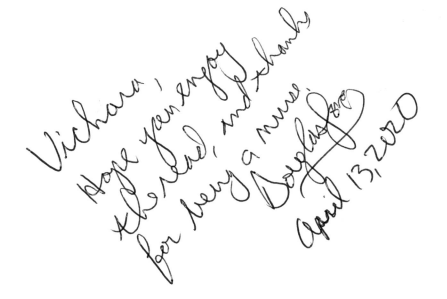

Vichara,
Hope you enjoy the read, and thanks for being a nurse.
Douglas
April 13, 2020

Nursing: Moving Forward by Douglas Long

To contact the author: NursingForward2020@gmail.com

Printed by Kindle Direct Publishing. Available from Amazon.com and other retail outlets.

First edition, January 2020.

ISBN: 978-1653442959

Contents

Preface

Nursing was not my first career choice. Nor was it a second or third choice. In fact, it is a testament to the vagaries of life that I ended up as a nurse. The story of how nursing became my profession and calling after many other twists and turns will also help explain my perspective on what nurses do and how we do it.

My prior career was in ocean shipping, sitting in a cubicle wearing a white shirt and tie, and setting the prices for containerized cargo crossing the Pacific. The shipping industry has almost entirely left the United States for Asia, and particularly China. Like many Detroit autoworkers, I found myself on the losing end of globalization. Nearing 40 years old, it was time to make a drastic choice.

I wanted a career that could keep me physically active, outdoors, and made a meaningful contribution to society—so nursing was not my next option. Instead, I signed up for the police academy and completed the six-month program. In the average police department, about 2 to 5 percent of all applicant get accepted; of the roughly 40 students in my class, less than half even graduated, and only a handful had already been hired and sent by their departments.

While my time at the academy gave me a new respect for law enforcement officers, and I learned first-hand just how rigorous is their preparation, even graduating did not assure me a job. In fact, my previous work in human rights and my messy state of affairs as a 40-year-old in career transition made it hard to land that first job.

So, I shifted my attention and took a class to become an emergency medical technician (EMT). On the first day of class, I teased three nursing students present about spending the rest of their lives wiping butts. That night I checked online how much EMTs make. No, that would not work. Paramedics? Still pretty hard to make ends meet on that salary. Nurses. Wait, how much do nurses earn?

Northern California has the best-paid nurses on the planet. The next day I returned to class, tail between my legs, and begged the nursing students for forgiveness. I asked them, please, to tell me what it takes to become an RN.

As soon as the EMT class was done, the first ambulance company to get my resume hired me. My first task was doing inventory of an ambulance, on a freezing cold winter morning in the parking lot. It could only get better from here, I thought. I would never be lacking for work again. I returned to my local junior college for the nursing prerequisites, then entered Samuel Merritt's accelerated one-year nursing program. After several months on the ambulance, I got into an emergency department (ED) as a technician and worked there until nursing school was done.

My first job as a registered nurse (RN) was in a local hospital emergency department (ED). Working in nursing was amazing and cool. There is no better way to describe it. We were in the center of daily drama, with lives in the balance. Even without the mortal risk, the personalities, challenges, and conflicts that played out in the acute care setting made me realize this was the perfect fit for me.

The job as a new RN in an entry-level position was hard. Every day seemed like a challenge to get all the tasks done. Still, there was a bigger problem brewing. Even with my total effort and having had a couple years on an ambulance and in the ED, nothing I did ever seemed good enough. There was constant conflict among the staff and with nursing management. What was going on? Things should run smoothly in a world-class hospital, but that was not happening. It was then that I began to think about the source of the problems, and to begin to imagine of a solution.

That is when this book began to take shape in my head.

I am very restless, physically and intellectually. There is no time, day or night, when my mind is at rest. Often, I'm thinking about theoretical things. To be called a nerd is, to me, a complement. Here I was in an ED with lots of smart people working hard but never accomplishing all that was expected of us.

I remember the manager calling me in once during a shift change to inform me of something. Then I walked out to take over patient care of someone being admitted upstairs to a medical-surgical unit. As I was pushing the patient in the gurney, another manager tagged along to see how I, a new RN, would handle giving a report as part of the hand-off. The report I gave was that the nurse on the prior shift had already left before I got onto the floor, and I knew nothing about the patient. I offered the documentation done by that other nurse. Any question, I asked?

The manager was shocked. She seemed to think it was my fault. Even she was overwhelmed in her role.

Some nurses have decades of experience in countless facilities, locations, and nursing specialties. I do not have that. Again, it's a second career for me. What I do have is an ability to compare nursing to other fields, to see where things are working well and where things are going wrong. I think it comes from a combination of things. For one, I am an outsider; 91 percent of nurses are female. But I also bring the experiences of coming to the career late, after doing other things— which isn't typically the case with the nurse I've met and with whom I've worked.

This book was written with the perspective of someone who is in the profession, still working in direct patient care, but with that outside perspective. My first attempt at documenting the problems I saw and the solutions I was beginning to imagine was very different from what you will read here. I began with a mental accounting system. What were all the things we nurses needed to do? The result was something like a list of "10 qualities of a good nurse," the sort of thing we sometimes read in trade journals. I realized that a good nurse needs to be several different people at the same time: a caring nurse, a physically fit nurse, a communicating nurse, and so on. My list eventually became seven aptitudes that a good acute care nurse needed to have. But that work on a book made me realize there was a deeper problem, and some more important points to be made.

I changed my direction—and that is what I hope you will choose now to go on to read. This book was written for nurses, to help move our profession forward. It should also be helpful to other healthcare professionals, hospital managers, and public policy makers. The issues I discuss are important if we are going to improve our community's healthcare system. That, and my desire to recognize the great work of my fellow nurses, is what pushed me to write.

While all the material here has research at its foundation, some of what you will read is presented with a more experience-based flavor. This is especially true of "On the Road" section of chapter 1, as well as chapters 6 and 7, which are the stories of my travels to nursing boards, regulatory agencies, and professional associations around the United States and throughout the world.

With one exception in the final chapter, every event I describe in this book happened, although in some cases I have changed the names and exact locations for the sake of confidentiality. If one of these events sounds familiar, it is almost certainly not that I am referring to your hospital, but it shows that these kinds of things are happening everywhere, and frequently.

All views expressed in this book are my own and do not represent the opinions of any entity whatsoever with which I have been, am now, or will be affiliated.

Acknowledgments

I have received extensive assistance and advice throughout this project, from the research and travel to the writing of the manuscript, and my heartfelt gratitude goes to all those who helped me. Space allow me to mention only a few by name whose contributions must not go unrecognized. John Bernhardt, who gave me extensive comments and keen insights, reviewed my first draft. The manuscript bears the mark of Suzanne Gordon, one of nursing's greatest authors, who despite her busy schedule found time to steer me in the right direction. Matthew Rothchild, a community activist and editor based in Wisconsin, worked on an initial rewrite. The single greatest change in the manuscript, in fact an entire recreation, came from Scott Cooper, based in Boston. He looked at what I was trying to say and led me through a process that rebuilt the entire book.

Among the nurses who have worked alongside me, Mariela Gomez, a nurse from Bogotá who is now at UCSF, distinguished herself in our nursing board visits worldwide. Hamza Alduraidi, my doctoral classmate, helped me throughout the Arab world research project and beyond. He has since been promoted within his university and, I am thrilled to announce, was finally granted a visa for Europe (a persistent problem described in chapter 6). Ia Gelenizhe has been pushing the nursing profession forward in her native country of Georgia, but still finds the time and energy to work with me on my research into nursing internationally.

Other individuals have helped me along the way in small but important ways. Jean Watson, a living legend (it's even on her business card!) in the nursing world, received an early version of the manuscript in which I heavily criticized her work and still invited me to join her for breakfast in Boulder, Colorado. In a world where people take offense at the slightest thing, or do not take time for people who do not seem important enough, she was open, honest, and receptive to my ideas. At the International Council of Nurses in Geneva, Switzerland, Alessandro Stievano opened the doors and let me in to learn about his organization. Cary McCarthy, an inspiring nurse trying to make a difference in a vast organization, introduced me to the World Health Organization.

This book would not have been possible without the intellectual tools gained in my doctoral program at the University of California, San Francisco. I would like to thank my advisor, David Vlahov, and my committee members, Abby Alkon, Heather Leutwyler, and OiSaeng Hong.

Finally, I would like to thank the many individuals that have helped but who here go unnamed. Some took risks by discussing sensitive topics. Others gave me precious time from their busy schedules. My hope is that their contributions prove to be worthwhile.

Douglas Long
San Rafael, California
January 6, 2020

Introduction

Sherry (not her real name) holds a special place in my heart as one of the best nurses I have ever had the honor to work with. She was an ICU nurse at San Francisco General Hospital for several years, and then transferred to Marin General Hospital where she was one of the key players in the Emergency Department (ED). Even when things were going crazy, she kept calm, her voice remained even, and she explained as much as possible to me even during those exhausting 12-hour shifts.

On one occasion, there was a psychotic homeless person fixated on her, spewing profanities and threats. Not in the least bit offended, she simply worked around this patient, walking the long way around the nursing station to avoid contact. She took no personal offense and understood that this was part of getting the job done when dealing with challenging patients. When a patient's medication list included some obscure drug no one else had heard of, she seemed to have the mental dictionary of a pharmacist.

One thing she said still stands out. A rather old nurse was working in the ED one day, and asked me, as a student, to start an IV and let a half-liter of normal saline drip in over the course of an hour. I did so, but forgot to follow up. The whole liter ran in. The older nurse pointed out my mistake and warned me to be more careful. I asked Sherry, why not just put the bag of NS on a pump? Why did that other nurse think it acceptable to let the bag drip when one might forget to keep track? She

1

said to me, "Don't ever question senior nurses." These words still repeat in my mind.

Nurses are almost unique in the number and variety of demands presented by their job. Other jobs require you to be smart, or to have a specific skill, or simply to show up on time and stay awake. Nursing, on the other hand, entails a set of demands that are highly diverse. The nurse must be smart enough to manage vast amounts of information, and this information must be processed and tasks carried out in a highly stressful environment. All the while, physical fitness is required because nursing is still a very athletic profession, and injuries are the single largest cause forcing nurses to retire early.

There is no standard list of a nurse's job requirements. Managers and employers struggle over this question. Job descriptions used in hospitals are a good place to start, and this gives us a first look at the problem. Hospital job descriptions for a nurse include multitudes of broad and vague demands, and the list often ends with a statement to the effect of "do whatever else we ask you to do." In other words, our employers are writing our job descriptions with no limits, giving them the option of demanding whatever they want of a nurse.

The nursing profession is not making the connection between all the disparate demands made of nurses and how they sum up to something unreasonable and unachievable. The challenge is not just the workload, or the stress, but all the diverse demands combined. Normally, when a person has a full workload, if you want her to do more of this, then you need to have less of that. You cannot simply keep piling on the demands and expect better results, but this is what nurses are being faced with.

Even if we can improve efficiency in some manner, demands are going to increase, and the problem is going to intensify. Innovations that might appear to ease the workload often only pile it on. One example is in documentation. The increased use of electronic health records has not reduced the nurse's workload. Quite the contrary. The workload has increased, and management's expectations have risen, as well. Nurses now have to track more data and make fewer mistakes. Although 99 percent of mistakes do not affect the patient, we still need to account for them because the event was captured in our documentation.

There is no endless supply of good nurses. Many people have a mistaken belief that if the person serving them, whether it be a waitress in a restaurant or the nurse in a hospital, is not good enough, there is a much more qualified person somewhere out there. It is just a matter of getting that subpar worker out and a better one in. The world is not like that. We hear of the nursing shortage, and the first solution that comes to mind is to increase the supply of nurses. How do we get more nurses? One way is to increase the pay.[1] Nurses are already the single largest staffing cost in any hospital, and Americans are paying far more for healthcare than any other nation, and the value added by nurses has been hard to identify. Even if we chose to offer more money, we are probably going to attract those who are more interested in the paycheck than the patient care. Another alternative is to provide more training, but that is also not a solution. Every increase in training is essentially an increased demand made of the nurse. If we already have a nursing shortage, and the training of nurses gets longer, tougher, and more expensive, these increased barriers simply reduce the supply of nurses.

Our society needs a large number of nurses, in every community, serving a variety of roles. This is not a small group of people, such as astronauts or police SWAT teams. There are about three million registered nurses (RN) in the United States—about 1 percent of the total population.[2] This is the essence of the problem: We need a large number of nurses, yet the demands placed on them are huge. This creates a strain on each nurse trying to fulfill the expectations placed on her. When these expectations are not met, patients suffer. Mistakes happen. Ultimately the nurse must face the consequences, which may be stress, injuries, disciplinary action, or even losing her job. If we only needed a small group of nurses, we might reasonably expect the best of the best. But if, as a society, we need a large pool of nurses, our expectations need to be realistic.

We nurses have not figured out what is a workable scope of practice for nurses, and what is an acceptable level of performance. The beginning of a solution, which I try to lay out in this book, is that we need to make some hard choices about what is most important. The next steps are to design the nursing role for success, instead of setting her up for failure. Education is a vital part of the process, before and during nursing school, as well as in the continuing education that seems to annoy us in our busy days instead of helping us do a better job. Vast amounts of resources can be wasted training for skills that ultimately may not add value, so I will target the skills that are crucial.

Along with the task of establishing a viable job description for the nurse is the task of establishing a viable way to assess her performance. That, too, is proving to be fiendishly difficult. My preceptor, Sherry, was an excellent nurse. It would not take a lot of effort for the ED supervisors to figure that out. However, she was once a new nurse, untested and unknown. All of us have been in that position. What if Sherry did not get along with someone and that person made accusations or complaints? One of the greatest challenges in nursing has been bullying, and that makes it extremely hard to separate legitimate complaints from frivolous ones. Any management system is going to lead to gaming, in which the nurse works the system to her advantage. This is normal human nature. It occurs when nurses avoid certain patients that are known to be difficult, or do not want to have their name on a patient's chart when things look bad. We need to create a system that acknowledges gaming instead of ignoring it.

Assessing the nurse's performance leads to the next step: making her face the consequences of her actions. This includes rewards and punishments, accolades or condemnations. Because nurses are licensed professionals, additional burdens are created because it is easy to coerce and discipline us. Not only do nurses face unprecedented job demands. We then get judged by anyone and everyone—from the patients to the employers, from government regulators to private lawyers. A common tactic of government regulators struggling to enforce a rule is to go after a person's license. The purpose of issuing a license is to ensure that only those who can provide safe care are allowed to practice. That license is not meant to be a leash that can be yanked back by any government authority on a whim. The nursing profession has not fought back against this practice. To the contrary, the argument is made within our ranks that a nurse is of such esteem that any of those offenses make her unfit to practice. Nevada's Board of Nursing provides an excellent example of nursing in the crosshairs (see the Appendix). Again, the nursing profession has not challenged this regulatory regime but actively encourages it.

When a nurse is accused of a mistake, her actions are judged based on these unrealistic standards. The legal standard is what a reasonably prudent person would do.[3] The problem with this is that we have lots of unrealistic standards, and the nursing profession keeps pretending as though these are realistic, while the actual level of performance by average nurses throughout our society is something far less. Nurses need to cut corners and manipulate the system to satisfy these disparate and unrealistic demands. Most get away with it because supervisors, hospitals, and government regulators know the system is dysfunctional and choose to let it go. When a nurse is facing discipline, managers do not investigate the mistakes her coworkers made. They only compare what she did to the mythical standards. We often hear that treatment and patient care need to be done so thoroughly that if anything ends up in court, the nurse has done everything properly. There seems to be some agreement among healthcare professionals that this results in bad practices and is illogical and unfair, yet we still do it. As a profession, nursing has failed to stand up to management that caters to lawyers rather than to good healthcare practices.

Consider an example of what every nurse does on a daily basis: the checklist. Every shift we tick off checklists for things like the code cart or medications. While some nurses diligently check every single item, it would be safe to say there are large numbers that do not. When inspections occur, those checklist forms tend to magically get filled up, as if they were done on every shift as required. Any time a nurse ticks off a box without checking, that is a falsification. Since problems almost never happen, there are usually no consequences. The point here is that nurses, supervisors, and the hospitals are living a lie, pretending on the one hand that these routine forms are vitally important, yet they can be falsified without consequence.

The Power of Nurses

Nurses are overworked and overwhelmed; yet the irony is that we have the power. It is within our profession to make the changes I propose in this book. I encountered repeatedly, as an outsider entering the nursing profession midcareer, nurses complaining about their job. You will not hear a lot of sympathy from me. It is not that I do not care about the need for us to take control of our profession. It is simply that we do not make use of the powers we have lying in plain sight. Three million strong, RNs in the United States constitute a major financial, organizational, and political force that cannot be ignored. Doctors have been at the top of the healthcare food chain, but there are not nearly as many of them. When you look at the quantity of nurses, and the amount of money we get paid, and the central role we play in the overall health outcomes of patients, nurses are the center of the healthcare system.

Nurses need to protect the profession and its reputation, which means being careful about who gets to be licensed as a nurse, and what is included in the job description. There are many who like to call themselves nurses, and a broad range of services could be referred to as nursing. The profession of *registered* nursing is much more specific and is specified with a government-issued license. It has been said that if you want to lead a parade, find a parade and get in front of it. Since nursing enjoys the public's trust, there are benefits to standing in front of this parade. Some nurses work in hospitals, while others have never worked in a hospital since nursing school. Others are in clinics, schools, prisons, or military bases. Some handle the critically ill, and some have a patient base of quite healthy people. Protecting the profession is no easy task, and egos run strong.

As we have heard time and time again, there is a nursing shortage. There is more than a mere shortage, and it is not wavering with periods in which supply meets demand. Society needs far more nurses in management and government. Unfortunately, the people running our healthcare system have virtually no clinical experience in any healthcare field. Vast areas of the world lack even the barest number of professionally trained nurses to meet their needs. More nurses are starting their career without ever having worked in any hospital, and there does not seem to be much concern about this. Even if we see a balance of jobs with nurses filling those positions, there is a downward trend in skills and experience. Nurses without basic skills are filling positions because of this nursing shortage. Even though nurses in the U.S. are the largest and most significant block of the heath labor force, that is still not enough to meet our needs.

Historically it has been doctors that enjoyed the credit and the power. In the past few decades we have seen a tectonic shift. Nurses are now becoming the central focus of healthcare after a history of having been seen yet unheard, admired yet disempowered. Doctors are expensive and nurses have been relatively cheap. This is why we do not spend money to have the doctors give routine medications or simple procedures. Nurses could do so much more than their traditional scope of duties. Gradually we have been taking on more and more of the thinking tasks, which are now referred to as "critical thinking." The more of these tasks that nurses took on, with great success, the more our jobs evolved.[4] Instead of a chasm of skills—and pay—between nurses and doctors, we now have a spectrum, not quite smooth, but definitely a spectrum. Whatever a doctor can delegate to nurses is getting delegated. We should not be sitting around waiting for our jobs to be delegated to us. We should stake our claim to them.

All of these demands are taking a toll on nurses. Job dissatisfaction is four times greater among nurses than that of the general public.[5] This is not just in the U.S. and not just a transient phenomenon. European countries reported that as many as 50 percent of them intended to leave the profession.[6] When nurses are not treated well, or when the demands of their job are too high, they vote with their feet, leaving the job, resulting in immense costs to the hospital. There has been a wide variation in turnover rates, to as much as 30 percent for new RNs, and a national cost to society of more than $2 billion. It costs upwards of $100,000 to replace one nurse.[7] Addressing the demands made upon nurses will then benefit not just the individual but also the patients, the hospitals, and the healthcare system. The good news is that we are valuable. The implication is that we need to offer our patients and our employers the service they need.

The nursing profession is at a critical juncture, still young enough that we have in our midst some of the pioneers that propelled the profession, but now trying to find a suitable role on the healthcare team alongside doctors and other clinicians. The future of nursing is going to include more community and home care. An increasing number of nursing graduates have never worked in any hospital. We need to sort out what is the nursing profession, its scope, and how to assess nurses and nursing in the most acute setting. This is where nurses traditionally have begun their careers and develop the skills that may then be applied in less acute settings, where the nurse is not going to get the experience needed to handle emergencies. The hospital-based nurses are working around many other nurses and health professionals, in a very rich learning environment. Once they are in the community, there is much less exposure to such resources. If we are unclear about how to manage the nursing profession in the hospital, things are only going to get worse when more nurses are in the community, so let's attend to this problem now.

The first chapter seeks to establish the premise that nurses need to take control of their profession, for the benefit of the patients and the nurses. We have major divides among us, such as management and labor, bedside nurses and advanced practitioners, and so on. Working together is not easy and not as obvious as it may seem. After that chapter, I address four topics that are among the most important in moving us forward. Nursing has been called the caring profession. There is much truth to that, because we aspire to something more than simply earning a paycheck. Nursing is the most trusted and admired profession, for good reason. However, that has allowed us to become sloppy about what it means to care.

The chapter on smarts seeks to make sense of all the information nurses are expected to absorb, process, and use in their patient care. Our job performance is based to a large degree on what things are considered important and what is not. Some nursing behaviors, such as caring, are hard to express as information. This chapter introduces a concept of smarts, which is information as expressed by nurses.

Medication errors, and mistakes in general, have had enormous influence on our jobs and, I will argue in that chapter, become the tool of choice for bullying. Having a "just culture" is an ideal we can realize, but not until we have come to grips with why we work in a profession defined by mistakes more than achievements.

Building on the previous chapter and its recognition of bullying, Chapter 5 shows how nurses use bullying to protect themselves as individuals, even though it undermines patient care and the nursing profession. If we want to work together as a healthcare team, we need to see bullying for what it is: a reaction to a dysfunctional incentive structure.

Finally, the last chapter offers specific recommendations based on the problems and opportunities I note throughout this book. There are many ways that we can take control of our jobs and the profession, and I enumerate them in this last chapter.

Introduction References
[1] Neal-Boylan, *The Nurse's Reality Shift*. She offers a variety of possible solutions, but is also realistic about their limits, such as more pay.

[2] National Center for Health Workforce Analysis, *The Future of the Nursing Workforce*. This report found 2.9 million RNs in 2012, expected to grow to 3.8 million by 2025.

[3] Guido, *Legal and Ethical Issues in Nursing*, 92.

[4] Garlo, "Critical Care Nurses."

[5] Aiken *et al.*, "Nurses' Report on Hospital Care in Five Countries."

[6] Aiken *et al.*, "Nurses' Reports of Working Conditions …"

[7] Li and Jones, "A Literature Review of Nursing Turnover Costs."

1

Nurses Take Control

New nurses are warned to try hard and be nice to everyone. I started my nursing career in a local hospital, after already having spent a couple years as an emergency department technician (ED tech), and as an emergency medical technician (EMT) on an ambulance. On the first day of my EMT class, which proved to be the start of my new mid-life career change into healthcare, the instructor made it clear what it takes to succeed. "That patient is having a crisis. It's his crisis, not yours. At the end of the day, you're going home." That told me that no matter what happens in the ED, I should remain calm and focus on what needs to be done. Surely I was prepared for my new role as an RN.

As it turns out, things were not that simple. Within a day, I had a patient having a reaction to the medication, so the doctor prescribed 25mg of Benadryl. No problem; this should be easy. It comes in 50mg bottles, and after I gave the prescribed medication, it dawns on me that the bottle was twice the prescribed dosage. What to do with my error? Fill out a report? Tell the doctor? No, that's all right. The Benadryl was to address the reaction, and the preceptor didn't think any harm would come of additional medication.

In nursing school, they taught us two things. Always report any errors, because the worst thing a nurse can do is lie. And get along with everyone. I do not recall my instructors pointing out the inherent contradiction.

The responsibility I had just assumed was not new. As a teenager growing up in California, I would spend my weekends in Yosemite National Park, the world's rock climbing destination, with my buddies. Here were a couple teens, still far from being adults, with our lives in our own hands. No parent was around to save us. No police or schoolteacher was there to tell us what to do. My partner depended on me to protect his life, and I depended on this scroungy 16-year-old guy to keep me alive. So, the responsibility that came with working in the ED was nothing new to me.

Still, there was a sense that something was not right here. As the first days and weeks in the new nurse orientation passed by, there was a trend appearing. Nurses would make a big issue of some mistakes, or even make up things to appear like a mistake. Yet other errors would go unnoticed. One day at the start of the shift, I was in the trauma room where the patient was on the monitor, and it did not look good. The RN assigned to work with me had me review the charts and check for new orders. I looked at the monitor and said, "should we report that to the doctor?" She never looked at the monitor, but said we needed to check for new orders. Missing a doctor's order is the worst thing we can do. She was annoyed that I seemed fixated on the monitor. Finally, an hour later, the doctor came in and sees the monitor. "How long has that been going on?" An hour? Why had I not told him? My buddy nurse just stood there, silent. What was going on here? This did not make any sense.

Those first months as an RN in a busy department are when I started trying to figure out what was going wrong with the staff and the hospital. Nurses were constantly scrambling to keep up. New patients were always appearing. Those already in the beds were presenting with new complaints, new crises, and new requests. Doctors would write orders, some of which were easy to accommodate but others never got carried out. Instead of working as a team, nurses were constantly on the defensive, fending off accusations, or working closely with others to cover for their mistakes. Instead of complaining about the workload, we simply trudged on. No one would simply say no this dysfunctional system.

Even if a nurse complained, supervisors were as overwhelmed as we were—or more so. They were on salary, and a 40-hour workweek usually meant 60 hours. The charge nurse was routinely cleaning beds to get more patients out of the waiting room, where wait times were closely monitored. There was a senior RN, the world's most overpaid bed cleaner.

The situation in my local hospital was not an exception to the rule. It was not an isolated event. At that time, I had already seen dozens of other hospitals because of my time on the ambulance. As an EMT, I would transport patients to and from almost every hospital in the San Francisco area. The daily scramble to keep up was being played out in every hospital on any day of the week. Holiday weekends could be counted on for an extremely heavy census, but any day could turn into a rush.

I also took the opportunity early in my career to become an American Heart Association instructor, first of Basic Life Support (BLS), then the Advanced Cardiac Life Support (ACLS). In every class were nurses, doctors, paramedics and other healthcare providers. This was a golden opportunity to learn what was going on in the other facilities. Barbers have that reputation for being on the receiving end of gossip. They cut your hair while you tell them about whatever is on your mind. I felt like one of those barbers. Running the megacodes in these classes, my students would tell me what was going in their hospital, or nursing home, or clinic. Almost everywhere it was the same, nurses struggling to keep up. It was not even just the nurses telling me the stories. The doctors, paramedics and others would describe essentially the same situations. Hospitals may differ in a lot of ways, but they all seem to share a struggle to keep up with demand.

The problem, as I identified it, unfolded before my eyes. Again, nursing was a second career for me, so my perspective was different. Nurses that had always been nurses seemed to accept the situation as normal. They' had never known otherwise. You work hard in the bedside world until you get to that point in your life when, with many years of seniority, you move to a department where the workload is more manageable—or you leave nursing.

Nurses did not create this situation. As every additional demand piles on, nurses either kept working, silently struggling to cope. Or they complained, to no avail. Or they simply did not follow the orders. Many assigned orders were not completed. If the managers want an explanation for why that order was not completed, the time spent explaining oneself could have better been spent on the other orders still pending.

If nurses did not create this system, who did? The answer, as best I can figure out, is no one—at least not purposefully. Our current healthcare system is the product of history, in which we as a society demanded healthcare and providers offered hospitals and other outlets to provide these services. Hospitals don't get to dictate how our national healthcare system is run. They struggle to figure out how to match resources with demand. Medical care is not cheap, and money is a limited resource. I find it hard to blame the hospitals when they make harsh decisions about wages, benefits, and the services provided to patients. The public, both healthy and sick, are struggling to pay for healthcare. The stage is set for major conflict, and nurses are in the middle. When asked how nurses got to this untenable position, I would say it was forces outside of nursing that led us here. I cannot point to any one person, or organization, or law.

The situation I just described is found in the United States. It applies to some other countries, but not all. Great Britain has a different system, in which there is one government agency, the National Health Service. Policies about the role of nursing are not the result of historical vagaries, but actively chosen. For example, there was a plan called Project 2000 to drastically change the training and status of nurses.[1] A nurse would now be considered an independent provider, accountable for her own actions and could not simply say she was following orders. The apprenticeship program was replaced with school training comparable to what we see in the United States. Some of the issues I am raising are the result of the lack of planning among U.S. nurses, but even in Britain, theirs is a work in progress. I also hear of them being overworked and suffering from the same problems as their American counterparts.

Set Up for Failure

As a profession, nurses have been set up for failure. There are a thousand things you can do wrong, leaving you vulnerable to being accused. Consider the assessment we are taught to perform on every patient coming into the ED. There is to be a head to toe check for any and all signs and symptoms of a problem. Then we ask the patients lots of questions about their lives, their concerns, medical history, and so on. Then there is the records check. What is in the patient's records? Now that we have electronic records, we can go back through years of excruciatingly detailed reports. Or there is nothing, and we need to figure out why we cannot find any record of that last hospitalization. And it goes on and on. I have not even begun to recount what the nurse is now expected to document or report to the doctor. Then begins the diagnosis, ordering or diagnostics, and treatments. Already, we can see what is theoretically expected of a nurse is impossible to achieve. Shortcuts are an absolute necessity.

The response is to protect yourself from accusations. Nurses don't talk about mistakes. That would be an admission of guilt. Nurses have to bully others to protect themselves. Meanwhile, we pick our friends who can be trusted to work alongside us without causing trouble. In other words, do not report mistakes. The network of friends and confidants expands out of necessity because we work with so many others. We cannot always have that buddy working next to us. That is where cliques and what we call mafias come in. It is normal human nature to band together. It does not take an anthropologist to tell me that extended networks of close associates play a valuable role in helping any person achieve their goals of hunting food, building housing, protecting one's family, or performing the job of a nurse.

In California, we often hear reference to the Filipina mafia. There are large numbers of nurses from the Philippines, and they have the reputation for banding together. This is only half the story. We all band together. One facility I worked in had a clique of wives and girlfriends of police and firemen. That was the EMS mafia. In another hospital in San Francisco, a gay mafia ran the ED. In my local hospital, I referred to the ruling group as the Rainbow Mafia. No, it was not the kind of rainbow you find on a gay pride flag. My gay friends jumped to that conclusion, which was incorrect. It was a group of senior nurses from all ethnic and social backgrounds who ran the ED for their professional safety. There was no dominant ethnic group here, just seasoned nurses struggling to cope.

One of the senior nurses from Marin General Hospital was in my BLS class. I remembered her from my days in their ED, first as an EMT, then as a volunteer, and later in a preceptorship. She was not particularly friendly or mean, but it was clear that she was part of the ruling class. I asked her about the recent changes at Marin General, in which they changed from being part of a major hospital chain to being an independent hospital. There have been a lot of changes along the way.

This hospital is known for their cliquishness, particularly the ED. She was complaining of the changes, the uncertainty, and what she perceived to be disorganization. I asked her about the tendency for those senior nurses in the ED to run the show, but the word "bully" was never mentioned. She concurred, saying, "Yeah, those of us that have been there a while don't like others telling us how to do things."

How did nursing management play into this system? My supervisors were also struggling to keep up. Their job description was likewise open to any and all demands hospital administrators dumped on their desk. And likewise, senior hospital leaders were in their position because they succeeded in meeting the demands of countless powerful interests. At no place could I find the source of the problem. It was everywhere, and nobody was particularly to blame.

In some professions, if you follow policies and procedures, you are safe. Not so in nursing. We have no shortage of documents telling us what to do, but that is the problem, not the solution. Nurses routinely hear the warning, don't do that or you will lose your license. I often hear nurses saying, "My license is at stake."

If you want to get a rich understanding of the professional landscape for nursing, observing nurses in hospitals and other places we work provides only part of the picture. In my nursing school program, the instructors kept talking about California's nursing board and how it "runs" the profession. The board decides what clinical things nurses get to do and what standards of conduct are expected of us. We were given an impression that a state board, in every state of the United States, is in charge of nursing.

That made me wonder: What is actually going on with these boards? I discovered that visiting nursing boards and observing how they do their work—erroneously described as governing the nursing profession in their states—is a seemingly endless source of insight.

I wonder how many nurses have ever been to any board meeting in their own states or in states where they don't work.

For obvious reasons, the first nursing board I visited is in California. It's where I live and where I received my nursing license.

So many times in nursing school and then in hospitals I heard "don't do this" or "don't do that" because the California Board of Registered

Nursing (BRN)* will take away your license. I wanted to know who these people were. How do they make their decisions? And most important, is it really that easy to lose your license, just over a simple mistake or a bad decision?

I attended three California board meetings over the span of a year. Lots of issues played out. Each meeting taught me something new. Because California is so large, and to give all nurses a chance to attend a meeting, the meetings are held in different locations throughout the state. My first meeting was near San Francisco. The next month, the meeting was in Los Angeles. And so on.

Those experiences convinced me that it was important to go to other states and observe their nursing boards. I wanted something to compare with my home state. It was my experience with California nursing board meetings that launched me on my travels to board meetings across the United States and overseas.

My first California board meeting, in October 2014, was a two-day affair held at a hotel in Emeryville, just across the bay from San Francisco. It was in a large room, with two hundred seats or more. I noticed that lots of the people in attendance, both men and women, were wearing suits.

The first day was largely devoted to presentations by nursing schools seeking approval for new programs or changes to existing programs and those pursuing their periodic reaccreditation.

The audience was large and there was lots of public participation. During an "open mic" part of the meeting, several people made comments or requests. A group of nurses from the California Pacific Medical Center in San Francisco, who worked in the labor and delivery department, came forward to appeal for the board's help in dealing with "bad management." The request was rather vague, and I wasn't sure the board could do much with it.

Another issue concerned whether paramedics should be allowed to decide not to bring a patient to an emergency room. Many paramedics end up with "frequent flyers" in their ambulances—people who need social services and not a precious ER bed.

---

* California's Board covers only RNs, so is called the BRN. Boards in other states also include LPNs and other licensees, so are more commonly called the Board of Nursing (BON).

I remember when I worked on an ambulance and we responded to a 911 call for a homeless man who "needed" to go to the emergency department. Our ambulance was a "backup" 911 provider, meaning that the primary 911 provider—the local fire department's paramedics—had already responded and was giving us this patient so their ambulance would not be tied up with a non-urgent patient.

When we arrived, the homeless guy was standing up and in no apparent distress. We were struggling to figure out why he had called 911. When we asked him what his medical emergency was, he thought for a second, and then said, "My face is red." It was "worrying" him.

As it turned out, his buddy had been sent to the hospital earlier that morning, and he just wanted to get together with him. Yes, his face was red—because he was out in the sun.

We had no choice but to take him to the ED, creating a large bill for the taxpayers, and a much larger bill at the hospital when they would have to assess him.

Paramedics in California have their own board; the nursing board does not regulate them. It was unclear how this power contest between nurses and paramedics would play out in this particular "hall of power" in Sacramento. One thing was certain: there were no paramedics in the room, at least none that spoke up. Those who did speak were all nurses and all uniformly against letting paramedics make the call of whether to bring someone to the emergency room. It was apparent to me that power and authority explained a lot about how these issues are resolved. Who has more political power, the paramedics or the nurse? I'm guessing paramedics will not win this one.

In any case, by the end of the first day it was clear to me that the California board was a big deal.

Many boards across the country have formal disciplinary hearings at their regular, public meetings. I've been at several. At this first visit to a California board meeting, I found what happened to be less a hearing and more like what I would call a "trial."

Most of the cases I observed at that first meeting and at subsequent meetings involved drugs and/or alcohol abuse, but other common scenarios were grossly incompetent nursing care, stealing, or diversion of drugs (that is, stealing drugs, but not necessarily for the nurse's personal use). What unfolded was nothing short of public humiliation of the nurses brought before the board. Some of them seemed well prepared and provided well-rehearsed statements. Others were a babbling mess. Nurses often broke down in tears. It took a few more state visits to realize that there was something very wrong about how these public disciplinary trials unfold.

Nursing schools had brought students to watch nurses in trouble face the board and be questioned. It was sort of like a "scared straight" program, but with a big difference from programs that, say, bring kids to jails to hear from prisoners. In those programs, the kids are participants, not just silent observers in an audience.

I don't know of any strong evidence that "scared straight" programs work. I don't know how bringing nursing students to disciplinary hearings affects them. I've never gotten any generalizable information from the couple of my coworkers who remember having gone through the process. What I do know is that only a tiny fraction of all nurses ever get official board discipline and so, for the vast majority of students, what they get from being in the audience is at best some general knowledge about how their chosen profession is regulated—but not much else.

By the time I attended my third California board meeting, I had a good sense of what happens. But there was an important change: they were filming the disciplinary cases. Nurses who previously had to defend themselves before scores of onlookers would now be humiliated well beyond the room, in videos posted on the board's website. Apparently, the only board member who protested this decision—saying it was "unnecessary and harassing"—was not a nurse, but a public member from the business community. No other board members spoke up.

On the Road

After California, I started traveling to other states, attending their board meetings. And, as you'll read in a later chapter, I began to travel around the world to see how other countries handle the nursing profession. (There's an entire chapter devoted to those trips later in this book.)

My first board meeting outside of California was the Washington board—it's called the Nursing Care Quality Assurance Commission—featured a guest speaker from North Carolina giving a presentation about "Just Culture"—the idea that has taken hold in the medical community aimed at getting past the "blame culture" of the past, and that is posited on the notion that we are all human and we should not be punished for "honest" mistakes (I discuss this further in chapter 4). It was my first encounter with the concept, and was perhaps the most important thing about attending that particular meeting. I took note of the fact that when a board member asked the guest speaker how to implement Just Culture when people are concerned they could be held liable for not reporting a mistake, the speaker had no good answer.

Another notable thing about the Washington meeting concerned food. The meeting was held in a community center far from any restaurants. There was a big lunch buffet laid out, but an announcement was made that only board members and staff were welcome to partake. That meant I had no choice but to drive all the way back into town to get lunch.

It turned out that the issue of food at nursing board meetings was to become somewhat of a recurring theme for me.

I needed to see more, in other states. So I visited Oregon.

When I attended a meeting of the Oregon State Board of Nursing, it was only the second such board I visited outside of my home state. So, I didn't have much with which to compare it. Nevertheless, I was tremendously impressed by the professionalism and competence—an impression that persists today even after I've traveled to board meetings across the country.

Let me tell you why. The evening before the start of the regular meeting, the board held a special session to plan for the next year and determine priorities for its special projects. The meeting was not only open to the public, but members of the public in attendance, about a dozen in all, were encouraged to participate. Board members asked me join them in this process. I deferred, explaining that I wasn't an Oregonian and was there as an observer of state nursing boards. I thought it would be inappropriate for me, an out-of-state visitor, to be influencing the process in any way. So, I sat back and watched.

To this day, I've been at no other board meeting in any state that invited public participation in this way. Nor have I seen any other board hold a special session to plan for the coming year.

Oregon wasn't the only big surprise. So, too, was the Texas Board of Nursing, which I visited some time later.

Many of us Californians have a stereotypical view of Texans as being simple, conservative, and not very friendly. Not so when it comes to the Texas Board of Nursing. In fact, I would say it ties with Oregon for most professional and sophisticated.

They say "everything is big in Texas," and that certainly fit for the meeting I attended. The room was big; the board members' upholstered chairs were huge; and the cop at the doorway was wearing one of those cool, big Texas Ranger hats. The attendees included a large group of nursing faculty and other stakeholders. They were all talking among themselves, but when they noticed me—someone they didn't recognize as being from there—they invited me into their conversation. I ended up being introduced to the board, and members asked me pointed questions about what I was learning from my research.

One notable thing about the Texas board is that it is one of the most ethnically diverse I've seen. In other states, most board members are white, and in some states the board composition do not come close to resembling the demographics of the nursing community or the state populace. Not so in Texas.

My Oregon and Texas experiences ended up informing a lot about what I think boards ought to deal with, and how they ought to look and function, everywhere.

When I visited the New Mexico Board of Nursing in October 2015, it was only the fourth such meeting in any state I'd attended. I was still "fresh" and learning a lot in every case.

The meeting took place in a massive conference auditorium at a hotel in Albuquerque. Board members sat on a table on a stage, far above the audience, much like in California. It was if they had positioned themselves to show how they imposed their authority over all. A few hundred nursing students were in the audience, there for the disciplinary hearings. Having come from the California meetings, which also had lots of nursing students in attendance, I thought public displays of discipline were the norm.

One case involved a nurse who came in with her leg on a rolling crutch. She moved slowly and her speech was slurred. She had been accused of being under the influence of drugs while at work. As she mumbled her way through her explanation, one board member asked, "Do you feel you are safe to work right now? If you had to go to work at this moment, could you do your job safely?"

"Yes," she responded. The audience gasped.

At hearing's end, she shuffled out slowly, a rather sad sight.

Next up was a male nurse, an ex-Marine, whose compliance with the disciplinary program was up for review. He was accused of not filing required paperwork—which he disputed.

A board staff member played the role of "prosecutor" and wanted to state for the audience the original actions that caused this guy to get into trouble. The nurse stopped the prosecutor right there, saying that was not to be discussed because mentioning those original actions would be embarrassing, irrelevant, and prejudicial. The only thing relevant, he insisted, was his current compliance.

In the complex rules of how these hearings are supposed to play out, there are times when you can ask questions (and only ask questions), and times when you can make statements or say whatever else you want to say. Under normal circumstances, this would be bewildering enough. But under circumstances where a person is defending his career and his good name while hundreds of people are watching, it's terrifying.

The "prosecutor" became upset at the nurse-"defendant" for not following the script perfectly: at the point in the process when the nurse was supposed to ask questions regarding his case, he instead made a statement defending himself. Finally, I thought—a nurse fighting back.

I thought the prosecutor was being a bully. Apparently, at least one board member seemed to agree with me, telling the prosecutor to back off because the nurse could not be expected to be familiar with the details of the process and should not be pushed around.

All this played out in front of the hundreds of nursing students. It was only later, after having been to many board meetings in which "defendants" were not subjected to public shaming, did I realize how the entire meeting was a travesty of justice from the beginning.

That same month, I went to West Virginia. The state has a reputation for being isolated from the outside world and for doing things its own way. I found that to be true. My visit to Charleston, the state's capitol, happened to coincide with that of another person—who came to talk about the opioid crisis. It was President Barack Obama. Luckily, the meeting of the West Virginia Board of Nursing was held on the outskirts of town and so wasn't affected by all the road closures.

By this time, I already had a pet peeve about state board meetings: the boards tend to set out a lunch buffet for its members and staff, and tell visitors not to touch any of the food. That's just rude! But in West Virginia, everyone was welcome to partake of what was an awesome spread. In the grand scheme of things, feeding meeting attendees is not important to the nursing profession. But as a gesture of hospitality, it goes a long way.

The West Virginia board was very cozy. Everyone at the meeting knew everyone else (except for me, of course). Members referred to nursing schools by the first name of the school's dean. Locals told me that sometimes the coziness meant personal connections and influence came before rules or qualifications. I didn't see anything to confirm or deny that assertion.

I did, though, observe an odd exchange between the board and the dean of the ITT Technical Institute's nursing program. ITT Tech, before it closed abruptly in October 2016—leaving tens of thousands of nursing students stranded around the country—was one of several multistate nursing schools. There has been an ongoing debate about the quality of instruction at these kinds of for-profit schools, and many think these schools are not up to the same standards as state and private nonprofit schools. In fact, when ITT Tech closed, many nursing schools welcomed the stranded students but would not give credit for any courses taken at ITT Tech.

The ITT dean of nursing was there to explain the schools low test-pass rates. Asked about how many of the forty states in which it was present ITT was on probation, she said she didn't know. I found that hard to believe. She was the head of all ITT's nursing programs nationwide, regularly attended state board meetings to address regulatory concerns, and claimed not to know that important piece of information? No wonder ITT's nursing programs had to close!

By this time, traveling to board meetings was becoming a very regular thing in my life. I began to plan ahead, laying out a schedule with the objective of visiting as many states as possible. My intention was to keep visiting different states to learn what was going on in the nursing profession. It was never my intention to visit all 50 states. These trips were taking a toll on my time, budget, and tolerance for jet lag and airplane food. In every state I visited, people I met remarked that it was the first time anyone had come from out of that state simply to observe a meeting, and none of the board members or attendees had ever heard of a nurse studying the boards as I was doing. That's what kept me going—knowing that this was a project worth doing.

In December 2015, I visited Nebraska. It's like other places in the Midwest I've visited, with lots of friendly people, little crime, and no problem finding parking—in this case, in downtown Lincoln, the capitol city. The Nebraska Board of Nursing covers both RNs and LPNs (the latter assist physicians and registered nurses with basic care such as administering medication, taking vital signs, collecting samples, addressing patient comfort issues, and reporting patient status). Board members at the meeting I attended were friendly, but as a whole they seemed disorganized—and as I began to think about why that might be, I realized there was a common thread among boards that struck me as disorganized: they are the ones that cover both these categories of nurses.

RNs and LPNs are, of course, all nurses, but they can be very different in terms of their scope of practice—that is, what they are allowed to do. That raises issues regarding how to regulate them, given that there will logically be different standards for different scopes of practice. The Nebraska board president was a LPN, and she seemed to struggle with being the chair. I wondered: if you cannot run a simple meeting, how can you regulate the nurses in your state? Most LPNs lack a college degree, for instance, and are often ill equipped to serve on a statewide board governing the nursing profession, particularly when most of the people in the profession have a higher level of education than that of an LPN.

The board raised an issue I was glad to hear addressed. A few years prior, I attended the meeting the National Council of State Boards of Nursing (NCSBN) holds each year specifically to discuss the National Council Licensing Exam (NCLEX). That particular year, it was in Calgary, Alberta. Canada. Every nurse in the United States and Canada needs to pass the NCLEX, and the cutoff score to pass is based on a complex mathematical system that involves a "logit"—something used to determine probability. Even I do not understand what exactly is a logit, and I survived a doctoral program with a specialty in quantitative research!

The Calgary meeting was a chance for the nursing community to learn about all the ins and outs of the NCLEX, and how the test is developed. I believe the complexity hides the fact that the people who create the exam just pick a point along a probability curve and decide, arbitrarily, that it will be the "passing grade" cutoff.

At the Nebraska meeting, board members were joking that they do not understand what a "logit" is—which was refreshing. I always appreciate when people admit they do not know something, especially if they are in a position where they should know. I saw this as a profound moment. It was the only board I have ever encountered with members who admitted they don't know what the cutoff point signifies other than a "passing grade"—in other words, they could not say what actual knowledge "passing" indicates.

Without getting into what ought to be used as a standard for passing the NCLEX, my point here is that the nursing profession is wrestling with complex issues that tax our collective abilities. Boards that include LPNs struggle to find anyone from that profession of nursing who are willing to serve, and those that do step forward are often ill equipped for the demands of the board position. This is another reason nursing professional associations and unions should be monitoring board activities closely.

At every nursing board meeting I've attended, I've learned something. Often, I get to see the very problems in my job in the ED play out across the country, and throughout the world.

The Nevada State Board of Nursing meeting I attended in January 2016 took place in a nondescript hotel conference room a block off the famous Las Vegas Strip. I sat in on what turned out to be one of the most dramatic displays of what needs to change in the nursing profession.

The meeting began with the public statement portion, during which anyone can step forward and have two minutes to say whatever. One local nursing professor asked the board to change the rule stipulating that a nurse admitting to a medication error is subject to punishment. Nevada's rule, she argued, was a violation of Just Culture, the concept I had first encountered at the meeting of the board in Washington State. Now it was being championed in Nevada—where, as it turns out, it is desperately needed.

Later that day, the board reviewed nursing schools for compliance with regulations. This, too, can get tedious—but not so in Nevada. The state dictates exactly how many students may enroll in a nursing program, and Chamberlain College of Nursing had admitted twice the number permitted. Board members seemed upset and wanted to know how that could have happened. Chamberlain had been given a clear and specific order, which the college seemed to have chosen not to follow. The dean of the nursing school was present, and she was told that her school was willfully violating a direct order. The board decided it would investigate why the school had admitted more students than allowed.

25

The Nevada board is not one to let any individual or any institution violate the rules, I thought. It turned out I was wrong.

The meeting continued the next day, when nurses came before the board for a variety of violations ranging from unprofessional conduct to stealing, and even arrests. One of the cases showed me, in vivid detail, why the nursing profession needs to change.

A licensed practical nurse (LPN, also known in some states as a licensed vocational nurse, or LVN) had been reported for unprofessional conduct. She worked in a home for children with developmental disabilities. One resident (patient) was a big, twenty-year-old guy who remained in a home designed for children because the insurance company was compensating the facility until he reached age 21.

This particular patient required parenteral tube feedings, which were made complicated by his tendency to lash out. One day, he was lying on the floor of the day room, where he liked to hang out. When it was time for his feeding, the particular LPN at the hearing came in to the room. There were three other LPNs in that day room; all of them were also at the board meeting. Her coworkers asked the LPN whether she needed help with the feeding.

"No, I can do this myself," she said. Typically, a few LPNs would be involved to hold his arms back and make sure no one got hit. But this time the one LPN straddled the patient and performed the feeding with no complications.

Or so she thought. It became clear from the board proceeding that this particular LPN was not getting along with her coworkers.

The other LPNs did not like the way she was straddling the patient, or maybe it was simply that they were looking for anything they could turn into a problem for her. One of them took a picture on a smartphone. They even contacted a supervisor. Notably, though, it wasn't one of the supervisors present in the facility at the time. No, they called another supervisor who was at home on her day off!

This LPN was now before the Nevada nursing board, accused of abusing a patient by straddling him while giving a tube feeding. She had come with a lawyer, who entered the room dressed so sloppily that I had a hard time believing he even *was* a lawyer.

The board was given the photo that had been taken, and they were not pleased. "Did they teach you to do this in your LPN school?" asked one board member.

The LPN's lawyer was ineffective, to say the least. To justify his client's actions, he actually said to the Board, "Well, shit happens."

There were so many issues at play. Let me explain why I said earlier that it was a vivid example of why the nursing profession needs to change. First, there's the issue of Nevada's code of professional conduct—which is long, detailed, and *vague*. I have seen no other state go to the lengths the Nevada board seems to go to detail, in its document, every possible offense for which they can discipline a nurse.

What I saw in the meeting was an LPN who was clearly being bullied by her coworkers being accused of abusing a patient just for adopting a particular physical stance while trying to provide patient care without getting beaten up. She was asked whether she had been taught to do that in her LPN school—but *no* nursing program, LPN or RN, goes into that kind of detail. We are taught to be adaptable and to improvise. And that is exactly what that LPN was doing.

As for her coworkers, the board had an admission, under oath, that they witnessed "abuse" and did not take reasonable action to stop it. If they believed that what they were witnessing qualified as patient abuse, why didn't they do anything to stop it? Instead, they took a picture and then chose to contact a supervisor who seemed to be their friend—and who wasn't even at work at the time.

In the end, the board found the LPN, who was just trying to do her job safely, guilty of patient abuse. This LPN was in school to become an RN, so that essentially ended her career as an RN and, possibly, as an LPN. I wondered whether the dean of Chamberlain College would get the same harsh treatment; after all, she had been told point blank that she had violated a specific order from the board. But a couple of months later, when the board next met, the minutes indicated that the mistake had been "corrected" and the Chamberlain issue was closed.

So, in Nevada, bullies prevailed and an LPN lost her career, while a nursing school acted with impunity and the dean apparently faced no personal consequences for ignoring the board's direct order.

What I witnessed in Nevada speaks volumes about the nursing profession. We have created a culture and regulatory system in which a nurse can be accused of almost anything. State boards do not consistently provide the clear guidance needed for nurses to follow, and thus the protections for nurses that come with that knowledge. Meanwhile, hospitals face enormous pressure to stay financially stable, and protecting nurses is not one of their priorities. When it comes to nurses, their focus is on the appearance of being "fair."

A Culture of Accusation—and the Stakes

We have created a culture and regulatory system in which any nurse can be accused of almost anything. Nursing Boards in each state do not provide the clear guidance and protection needed for nurses to follow. Hospitals are facing enormous pressure to stay financially stable, and protecting nurses is not one of their priorities. If it is a priority to a hospital, it is not to defend the individual nurse's interest *per se*, but to appear to be fair.

At this point, I have to ask: How did we get here? What does this say about the nursing profession? And just as important, where do we need to be heading as a profession? I just mentioned that the current situation is a result of historical processes and outside forces. Professionalized nursing has a relatively short history compared to medicine or other fields, so we need to give credit to our nursing leaders that faced a patriarchal world determined to keep nurses as quiet, obedient handmaidens. The good news is that we've been on a strong trajectory of growth, both technical and in terms of the authority wielded in the halls of hospitals and government.

Nursing scholars Suzanne Gordon and Siobhan Nelson have described how we are holding ourselves back as a profession by sticking to what they call a "virtue script."[2] We enjoy widespread respect and empathy from the public, which is a great thing to have. However, we are holding ourselves back by emphasizing the caring part of nursing while minimizing ourselves as knowledge workers. It is as if there was some conflict between the two roles. There is not a contradiction. What I saw as the problem was that we work under an unworkable set of rules, thinking that compassion and caring will make things OK. Instead, I argue that we need to continue this trajectory of professionalization by working together, nurses and nurse managers, in hospitals and in government. Instead of being in denial about unworkable rules and unreported errors, we need to acknowledge what is a workable job description. Nurses need the authority they desperately need to make the job workable.

What's at stake here is more than just nursing. The health and safety of our patients and the community depend on us getting this right, or at least better than what we have. As you will see in later chapters, information about medication errors is fundamentally flawed; nurses face retaliation for making innocent mistakes. Communication within nursing circles and with the rest of hospital staff is usually stifled out of concern for one's job and credibility. There are approximately three million RNs in the United States, which is about 1 percent of the population. Imagine you live in an average-size town of 100,000 people. That means there are a thousand nurses in your town. Put in those terms, and you see how important we are to our communities. Even if we do not enjoy the prestige of the doctors, nurses are central to our healthcare system.

Where was the union during all of this? Labor unions play a key role, protecting the nurse so that she can be the patient's advocate against others with different priorities.[3] Many states have little or no unionized nurses, and that, as I argue throughout this book, is dangerous. A nurse that cannot speak out for fear of retaliation cannot protect her patient. There is a fundamental inequality in which the nurse, by herself, is powerless against a hospital, which is a large and influential organization. And hospitals write policies that are far-reaching and vague, which gives administrators and supervisors the power to force or not enforce the rules, based on convenience, whim, personal grudge, a bad night's sleep, or any number of other factors, including a nurse's union activity.

Take one small example of how nurses need to band together. When you get hired, hospitals make you sign a form that says the information system will only be used for work-related purposes. No exceptions. Yet virtually everyone uses the Internet to check their personal email, news, and so on. It is difficult to write a policy that permits some common-sense approach to Internet usage, so we live with this grey zone. Unions are what bring common sense and reason to the process. There are role models for effective teamwork between labor and management. Kaiser Permanente has a labor-management partnership that serves as a role model for its deep and effective resolution of conflict, creating an environment where nurses contribute to quality improvement.[4] Tragically, many nurses in the United States and worldwide work in facilities where their talents are ignored and they are deprived of a say over their work lives.

The lack of union membership may be explained, in part, by our odd understanding of where we stand in the healthcare industry. Nursing is considered a profession, and we like to think of ourselves as professionals, much like doctors or lawyers. We do not want to think of our relationship with supervisors, managers, and leaders as confrontational. We are all nurses, working for the common good of the patients. One the one hand, we consider ourselves professionals, yet on the other hand organize ourselves like a blue-collar labor force, dividing rank and file from management. Unlike doctors or lawyers, a nurse cannot operate independently. She cannot hang out a shingle and set up her own practice. Regardless of how much we want to think of ourselves as professionals, we are more like regular workers. This should not be a problem. We can still be professionals *and* work together as organized labor.

In my journey to make sense of this all, I was noticing four major themes. The problem was that nurses have all the responsibility without the control to make it workable. It would be helpful to be more specific about what is being demanded, how it's not workable, and what we need to do to make this better. The first theme is *caring*. Nursing is the caring profession, as I have heard *ad nauseum*. I am not one to be overly sentimental. But I do care. That is why my life has been taken over for these past years trying to find a solution to the nursing profession's current situation. The kind of caring we are hearing about is best represented in Jean Watson's call for "loving," "intimate," and even "spiritual" relationships with our patients.[5] What started out as a perfectly reasonable expectation—a nurse should care about her patient and her professional performance—has turned into something else, and it is not helping us.

The next major theme is *information*, which comes at us from every direction, while we're expected to remember stuff, know things, and document facts at an ever-blinding pace. I refer to the way nurses handle information as "smarts." This is information as experienced by and managed by nurses in a real world clinical environment.

The third theme has to do with *errors*. Nurses are almost never rewarded for doing a good job, but are punished for making an error. A salesperson is rewarded for every sale he makes. At the end of the quarter, his boss does not really care about all those customers that did not buy anything. In other words, a salesperson is not judged on errors. Nurses can only do wrong. This is one of the things that need to change. There has been a lot of attention to this, as we can see from the frequent mention of *Just Culture*. But much more needs to be done.

By my estimate, the number of errors being committed by nurses is many times greater than even the highest estimates. Hiding those mistakes is why we have *bullying*. Nurses need to protect themselves, and that means working with people they can trust and getting rid of coworkers that are going to report every mistake.

For all those nurses that cannot understand why they are being singled out, you are not alone. I propose that we recognize bullying for the defensive mechanism that it is and create a more manageable nursing workload where there is no need for the negative behaviors. Teamwork means working with people that you do not necessarily like but have a common understanding what it takes to provide great patient care.

I have some specific recommendations based on the themes of caring, smarts, *Just Culture*, and nursing solidarity in the final chapter.

Chapter 1 References
[*] Bradshaw, A. *The Project 2000 Nurse.*
[2] Gordon and Nelson, "An End to Angels."
[3] Manthous, "Labor Unions in Medicine."
[4] Kochan *et al., Healing Together.*
[5] Watson, *Human Caring Science.*

2

From Caring to Professionalism

Florence Nightingale holds mystical status for her selfless devotion to caring for patients. That may very well have been her sole motivation, but look at the bigger picture of the role she played. When England was losing the Crimean War and countless soldiers were dying on the battlefield, she was helping the war effort by caring for England's wounded, while being credited for her selflessness.[1] Imagine if she put her efforts into caring for the soldiers on the other side of the conflict. It always struck me as ironic that nurses working for the military are considered caring and non-judgmental, all the while helping their nation win in the battlefield. The Hippocratic oath states that we are to do no harm, yet our services to the military help soldiers do their job of killing, often by getting them fixed up so they can return to the battlefield.

The point is not to lessen Nightingale's contributions, nor to criticize the military. Before I entered the nursing profession, I was proud to have served my country as an infantry officer. The point is to show how nurses get less guidance from the concept of caring than we have been led to believe. As nursing scholars Gordon and Nelson noted, we tend to lessen our knowledge and professional contributions in order to follow the caring script. However, caring matters because what we do as nurses matters—a lot.

Caring is the one defining word that has captured the image of nursing. The profession is dominated by this concept. Throughout all the changes over time and across borders, nurses are known for their caring attitude. There is something distinct about nurses that sets us apart from anyone else, hard at it may be to define. Some are attracted to this profession for just this reason. When the public was asked what they think of nurses, the first word that came to mind was "knowledgeable" (17%), and next was "caring" (16%), followed by "hard working" (12%).[2] (The sample included approximately 15,000 RNs and 1,600 members of the public.) Notice the profound sense of respect held by the public of nurses. The point is clear: Nurses are special. Given the significance of this for the nursing discipline, we need to understand what it means, what it does for nursing, and where it can take us.

The answer is far from clear. "Caring" is not well defined, and the word alone offers little guidance moving forward. To the contrary, our overuse of caring as a motto has allowed the nursing discipline to avoid facing some of the realities of the profession, which will create greater confusion in the near future. Good intentions and lofty ideals do not always help the nursing profession. Caring does not give nurses as much guidance on how to do their jobs as many have suggested. Recall Lisa in the previous chapter, who was found guilty of patient abuse. From what I could see as that tragedy unfolded, she was trying to care for a patient in a hostile work environment. Even if her behavior was unacceptable, it was not based in malice or laziness. In her case, caring did not help her much. By contrast, in countless other states, board members told me of how they asked nurses that had made a mistake, what were you thinking? If there were honest and caring motivations behind an honest mistake, the consequences were vastly different than if a nurse was simply trying to serve her own selfish interests.

The situation was not always like it is today. Nursing scholar Angela Williams describes how historically nurses maintained a detachment to deal with the intimacy of working on the bodies of strangers.[3] Then there was the "new nursing," which brought organizational changes that redefined the nurse-patient relationship, including the suggestion that the nurse should build a personal relationship with the patient. This has evolved to the point where nurses are being asked to care with their heart and soul, treat patients like family, and even have spiritual connections.

I think we have gone too far and left common sense behind. Instead of the "caring" that is vague and often ridiculous, we should describe our work as *professional*. There seems to be resistance to the term professional, as if it implies business and money rather than human value. That is one thing holding the nursing profession back and contributing to the overworked and over criticized nursing.

While much of this discussion sounds highly critical, the overall message is quite optimistic and positive. Caring behaviors can be found almost everywhere and are performed by people regardless of their intentions or feelings. Organizations can promote caring practices, so workers can demonstrate these higher ideals regardless of what they may be feeling inside. Nurses do not have a monopoly on caring. The good news is that there can be a *professional* caring.

I need to address several questions. What is caring, in terms of an aptitude of nurses? In other words, how do you know it when you see it? Is it something unique to nurses? Does it come with the job, or do all people have some degree of caring? What can we take from this ill-defined notion of caring to help solve the problem of overworked nurses? Regardless of what terms are used—caring or professionalism—we need to take responsibility for our work. But we are creating unrealistic expectations of ourselves.

What Does "Caring" Mean?

Definitions of caring tend to be long and vague, which should lead us to suspect that something is amiss. Nursing scholar Ora Lea Strickland referred to caring as something that "may be viewed as an attitude, an ability, an attribute or characteristic, or a complex of interrelated behaviors."[4] The statement that Jean Watson makes that comes closest to a definition may be that "caring is often considered an ethical worldview, an ontology, an intentionality, a consciousness, a way of being..."[5] Watson is something of a one-person nursing-related industry, with a long list of books and articles, cited by everyone who has anything to say about caring. She began her career using the term *caring*, but has since developed her own concept of *caritas*, borrowing the Latin term for virtue or charity and redefining it specifically for her idea of nursing. At the same time, her treatment of caring has evolved to include love and spirituality. For example, the 1979 version of the carative factors included "helping," whereas in the 2008 version it was described as "sustaining a loving, trusting, and caring relationship." The carative factor of what she calls "existential-phenomenological-spiritual forces" stretched into "opening and attending to spiritual, mysterious, unknown, and existential dimensions...."

Given Watson's iconic status in the nursing community, I felt it worthwhile to seek her out, which I did while on a trip to Denver for Colorado's board meeting.

The Colorado Board of Nursing meeting I attended took place in a high-rise office building in downtown Denver, in a room that was about four times larger than needed. It was an odd contrast to the meetings I've attended in many other states that jam everyone into small rooms.

That meeting was also the first meeting of a new board member. Another board member took time, as part of the meeting, to explain publicly to her how things worked. By this time, I had been at enough meetings of other boards to know what was about to happen: a board member showing up without any real preparation was going to be voting on issues that could profoundly affect the state's healthcare system or the career of individual nurses who appear before the board.

It reminded me of my visit to Nevada's board, when one of the LPN members was also new. There were votes that day on important issues, and some of those votes were split. That meant the outcome hinged on one member who was making his decisions without having any board experience. Sure, every board at one time or another will have to deal with new members, but some states seem to make the lack of preparation more obvious than others.

Colorado's board, like most others, spent some time reviewing the NCLEX pass rates of nursing schools. One school had a pass rate of 83 percent; a board member told the school's representative, "I want to see you at 100 percent"—which was followed by an admonition: "Testing. Testing. Testing." It was the same with every board: higher test scores were equated with being safer nurses.

But whether passing the NCLEX tells us whether an applicant is going to be a safe nurse is an open question. I know of no research that has attempted to match NCLEX scores with nursing performance. When I asked Doyoung Kim, the NCSBN senior psychometrician responsible for NCLEX development and testing, whether there had ever been a test of the outcomes, he replied that such research project would be impossible because the data are property of each state.[6] The

36

fact is that while the NCLEX exam itself is the property of the NCSBN, the results—including applicant demographic information and test scores—are owned by each state board. That's the case even if the applicant who takes the exam in one state came from elsewhere and plans to apply for a license in another state.

Kim's answer notwithstanding, though, there's no insurmountable obstacle preventing a state from providing data for research purposes. A researcher would need to determine what measure of performance to use, which raises how to define nursing knowledge and recognize it when it is being demonstrated, as well as what constitutes "competency." Research of that sort could be among the most valuable of any ever done about nursing, because it would have to include a concerted effort to identify all the current practices currently of thousands of nurses nationwide, which would constitute a consensus of nursing practice.

I guess, though, that's for another time. Back to the Colorado meeting.

Sometimes, a board gets into a deep discussion of issues related to nursing that help them solve a general class of problems but that are not directly related to any case before the board at that moment. When I've witnessed such discussions, they provide a glimpse into how the individual board members think. My first encounter with this had been in Oregon, where the board convened a special meeting the evening before the regular meeting to have just such a discussion. This happened in Colorado, too, although not in a special meeting.

The Colorado board's discussion—which was strictly hypothetical—was about patient abandonment. A scenario was offered: a triage nurse steps away from the desk when there is no patient there. If one is a triage nurse and does not have a patient at that moment, does walking away constitute abandonment? It was an interesting question.

The nurses on the board thought not, but the board's public member was very strict, and said it was like abandoning the patient. That the public member took the hardest line was no surprise to me; I had encountered a couple of other cases in which public members seemed to take very tough stances against nurses. It was yet another case of someone sitting on a nursing board who had thought about an issue a lot more than the average person and who in this instance pushed for the strictest interpretation of patient abandonment. Of course, he had never worked as a nurse.

That discussion reinforced for me an argument I've been making throughout this book: nurses are held to unrealistically high standards.

On that trip, the session adjourned early, giving me most of the day to explore. My first destination was Columbine High School, a place that haunts our collective soul as a nation. It had been 18 years since the infamous day, and we were still struggling to figure out how to solve these school shootings.

Part of my quest to understand caring is to explore the opposite, best exemplified by what happened in this quiet suburb. Once at the high school, everything appeared normal, except for the empty sheriff's car parked out front. Beside the school is a community park, and in the back, you will find a memorial to the twelve lost lives. It was very touching.

Think of the nurses that were working on the day of the shooting. They had dying children in their hospital, shot down while in school. If the two shooters had survived, they too may have been in that same hospital, being cared for by the same nurses. This conflict plays out every day, in which nurses are being asked to provide lifesaving care for the worst of society, without showing any resentment or judgment.

From there, I drove north to Boulder, a college town and home to the Watson Caring Science Institute, to meet Jean Watson. My phone app directed me to an office park. Is this the right place? I walked up to the building that was supposed to be the Institute, and on the wall was a listing of attorneys, and a few financial advisors. No mention of Watson or caring here. I walked in, and the smartly dressed front desk staff asked if they could help me. "I'm looking for the Watson Caring Science Institute," I said. She asked if I had an appointment. No, I did not. "Oh, well they normally only see people by appointment." OK, my question was answered. This was one of those office for rent outfits. This incident struck me as odd because I was expecting something warm and welcoming, but not in a professional and corporate sort of way. Then I remembered how I as a nurse work in hospitals, which are sterile, corporate things. It is the nurse's job to make it welcoming.

Despite that I have criticisms of some of her ideas, Dr. Watson has provided encouragement and input to me. She devotes her life to making a positive contribution. I have the utmost respect for her and appreciate her work. On the one hand there is Columbine and this horrible violence being played out time and time again while we fail to make the hard choices to control gun violence. On the other hand, you have Watson who wants us to be more caring and has devoted her life looking for ways to make that happen. My concern is that nurses struggling to keep up with the stress and workload of patient care are not well served by this current notion of caring as something loving and spiritual. Watson made herself famous by hard work, and organizational skills, which leads her to use a shared office. Nurses should use caring as a source of empowerment, but should not feel guilty for not achieving a goal that is vague and elusive.

Caring's Basic Conflicts

I was working in a pediatric emergency department in San Francisco, a big change from my prior job at an all-ages ED, where you have the young and old, but mostly the old. They are the ones that tend to have more healthcare needs. If you want to get good at nursing children, you need to work in a dedicated pediatric facility, such as this one.

One thing I hear a lot from pediatric nurses is that they love working with the children, but it's the parents that create the problems. So true. I was taking a few minutes to eat, and the nurse's break room is directly across the hall from one of the patient rooms, where a mother was sitting with her sick infant. She hit the call light. Even though I was on a break, I put the pizza down, and walked over to see what she needed. A binky. Sure, I can get that for her. A short while later, having eaten but not enjoyed that pizza slice, I was in her room trying to get an IV in the child. No success. As any nurse knows, you win some, and you lose some. Another nurse was able to get the IV in. A few days later I was called into the manager's office and told there was a complaint. I had not washed my hands when getting the binky, and I had failed to get the IV in. That other nurse—described as "a professional"—managed to "get the IV in on the first try." Interesting how she used that term "professional."

What is the nurse to make of all this? Let us step back and begin with the basics. Caring about something can mean two things. The first is the obvious: that you have an attachment, love, or appreciation for that person. The second type of caring is the recognition that something is important to us. The average person does not care much for gasoline. It is smelly, dangerous and expensive, but he does care about it because without it, his car will not run. This is the indirect caring, also known as instrumental caring. Think of your relationship with your co-workers.

You might feel a sense of camaraderie with them, but you need a job and you need to be there every day to earn an income. Now think of the co-workers that have left that job. How many did you ever hear from again? In nursing, how much of the caring behaviors are based on sincere and deep commitment, and how much of them are based on what is required of the job? You can care about the patient because this is a person for whom you have empathy, or you can care because it is your job. And, of course, you can do both.

Caring can also be that observed by others, and that which is felt inside. Behaviors associated with nursing services are called nursing care, or patient care. These are actions, independent of what may be going through the nurse's mind. Then there is the feeling, or motivation, of caring, when the nurse is motivated not by the salary but by the sense of doing the right thing for this individual. Nursing scholar Ann Bradshaw warned of the "McDonaldized" nurse: "The appearance of compassionate care will be nothing but a façade, a pale imitation, even a parody, of the former understanding of care as arising out of virtuous character."[7] Sociologist Arlie Hochschild, in her book *The Managed Heart*, coined the term emotional labor, in which people act as if they are caring, happy, or friendly because that is what the job requires.[8] There are a vast number of workers in this market for emotions, so nurses are far from special in this matter. Hochschild describes surface emotions, which are simply an appearance and nothing more, and 'deep acting,' which entails forcing oneself to feel whatever emotion is required through such methods as imagery or prompting.

Looking back at the experience with the binky, the pizza, and the IV that I did not get inserted, what was the role of caring here? I find that nurses who get the most credit for caring have mastered the art of fulfilling patient expectations. That means managing expectation and controlling risk. Some patients are going to be difficult. Best leave that one to another nurse, preferable the registry nurse who is not going to be around for very long. In this case, I could have shut the door to the break room so that she never knew I was there in the first place.

For Tonya Battle, it would not matter much what she did, because she was black. She worked in a Michigan hospital, in the labor and delivery room, and is held in high regard by coworkers and the hospital. One day, she looked at a patient's chart, and in there was a sticky note stating, "no black nurses." The father of the patient and child had, reportedly, asked that no black nurse handle this white baby. This father was reported to have a swastika tattoo. The case was settled out of court, so many of the details are not known. It is unclear if the patients had asked for no black nurses or if one of the other nurses had made that note out of concern that putting a black nurse with that patient would be problematic. What Tonya did tell me, via her lawyer, was that she respects all of her patients as equals and does not see color. All children are the same, in her eyes. Imagine her frustration at knowing that no matter what she does, at least one patient has already deemed her unfit, in his eyes.

As I think about this case and what we can learn about caring, it strikes me as tragic that we don't know about the details that could give us better guidance in handling situations like this. Workplace discrimination is usually condemned. However, when a patient requests something that may be considered racist, the guidance is often vague. One manager told me her hospital would not comply with any request based on "hate." Okay, but how does one decide whether that patient is hateful, fearful, misguided, or even reasonable? I as a male in nursing, have been discriminated against, but is that hate?

As a nursing student, I was in a medical-surgical unit clinical rotation in San Jose when a male patient—a new admission—was wheel-chaired in. Seeing me for the very first time from 10 paces away, he proclaimed loudly, "I don't want him in my room. I ain't gonna have no male nurse touching me. I ain't from San Francisco!"

The first rule of nursing, we were taught, was to ask questions. Clarify what the patient means by that. In this case, there were no questions asked. He simply got female nurses. If Tonya's patient had made the request, it may have been rejected, or it may have been accommodated in the name of safety. Putting a black nurse in a room with someone with a swastika tattoo is probably not the wisest thing to do. But these issues are guided in part by caring, but mostly by professional clinical judgment. Nurses as knowledge workers can get a better answer than simply to say we should love our patients unconditionally.

I see nurses being told that we must feel these emotions, in a work environment that is already at a breaking point of stress. It is not even clear to me that feeling these emotions are even necessary. There is little indication that others can tell when that worker is doing it simply for the

41

job or if they are feeling that emotion. When you see a person behaving in a certain manner, you infer why he is doing that and what is going through his mind. You observe a voter voting for a given candidate and think, "He must like that candidate." Then you realize there are a lot of other reasons the person is voting that way, many of which have nothing to do with the voter liking the candidate.[9] Maybe that candidate was only slightly less obnoxious that the other candidate. Even if the nurse tried to demonstrate her feeling of caring for a patient, that is not always going to succeed.

The opposite is also possible, in which the nurse appears to be caring but is not. Consider one famous case of a nurse who was described as a good nurse, but the reality was far different. Charles Cullen was a nurse who turned out to have a dark side, a very dark side, and he masked that dark side with caring behaviors. While working in multiple hospitals, he was killing patients through such means as over sedation and putting insulin in IV normal saline bags. We have no way of knowing how many people were harmed by his efforts, but he may be one of the most prolific killers of the century. When his coworkers were asked about him, the response was quite uniform. He was a good nurse.[10] Apparently, he was able to demonstrate caring behaviors to the satisfaction of a large number of people.

Demonstrating caring behavior is not the same as taking good care of your patient—that is, attending professionally to his clinical situation. Is it really necessary—or even possible—to always develop that "caring relationship"? Or is it OK to settle short of that? There is the "as if" principle, in which we assume that a person is acting "as if" they know what they're doing or their motives are decent. We recognize that "as if" may not be the right answer, but it is close enough. As nurses, we usually do not know much about our patients. We are assigned a patient, we go into the room and make an assessment of the medical issue, and moments later may have forgotten about him. But we are actively and dutifully caring about him. We are acting "as if" we care about him. The nursing world can accommodate that just fine. We do not need to truly care about the person in some profound way, but as long as we are acting as if we care, and as long as we utilize our professional expertise appropriately, we are doing what we need to do.

Another problem with the overemphasis on caring is that it provides a phony sense that nurses don't care about their compensation. If caring is a matter of personal commitment, then one would need to explain how it is that nurses make a generous living, yet we are somehow not doing it for the money. It is rather disingenuous to say one is doing this for the benefit of the patient, and that the paycheck is simply irrelevant or incidental. The relationship between the patient and the nurse is one of a customer paying a service provider. And yet many nurses and aspiring nurses downplay this basic relationship. Students were surveyed about why they picked nursing as a career, and the most common motivation, according to the students in their own words, was altruism.[11] Doing something unilaterally with no compensation can be considered altruistic. Doing something for others and receiving intangible rewards can also be considered altruistic. Yet nurses are paid for their services.

Job satisfaction among California's nurses has been increasing over the past years.[12] Contributing to this improvement was "quality of patient care" and "interaction with patients," suggesting that the caring factors matter. However, salaries increased from $63,000 to $85,000 in just four years. This is quite remarkable. The average nurse in California is earning 40 percent more than the average household income in that state,[13] yet "interaction with patients" was listed much higher as a source of satisfaction. The nurses taking this survey were not asked to make a choice between patient interaction and salary. There is no cost to say that one values patient care more than that generous salary. It is easy to take for granted an income that is essentially double what others with a similar education level are making.

Look at the pattern of nurse employment, and a trend is clear. Nurses move from areas of low pay to areas of high pay.[14] Florida experienced a nursing shortage at a time when large numbers of nursing school graduates in other states could not get a job. One explanation was the low pay offered in Florida.[15] One does not see large numbers of nurses moving to those areas where wages are low. There are exceptions, such as a nurse who may have family connections, is following a spouse, or is trying to get that first job and experience. A major trend in our field is the movement of nurses around the world, and it is invariably from the poorer countries to the richer countries.[16] These nurses leave behind family and community, and a society with fewer nurses, to provide for people who are much richer than the patients in their country of origin. This is not to suggest these nurses are insensitive to the needs of their own loved ones. Quite the contrary, they are typically doing this to better provide for their families.

The point is that money drives the movement of nurses, not some vague sense of caring for their patients. A hospital seeking to attract the best nurses must offer competitive salaries. It has been said that if you pay peanuts, you get monkeys. If you want the best talent, you pay the best wages. This does not mean that other factors, like working conditions, do not matter. But it begins with the pay. Overall, caring and uncaring nurses alike are seeking the best compensation.

Money and profit are held in disdain by some nurses because it conflicts with their notion of caring. We can see this in another way, as we are constantly hearing about the evils of hospitals that only want to profit while compromising patient care.[17] Hospital managers and nursing leaders are criticized for pursing financial goals, while providing no alternative for how they might be run. And while the profit motive undoubtedly at times runs counter to patient care, nurses themselves have actually benefited from hospitals' obsession with the bottom line. Hospitals run on money, not good will. Nursing professionalism has come about not by a group of nurses who randomly decided one day they wanted to be the equals of doctors. Those "heartless" hospitals worked with nurses to promote professionalism. Doctors made large salaries, and nurses made low salaries. It made sense to train nurses a little more and let them do some of those things doctors were doing at much higher salaries. The nurses and hospitals both gained. There has been an ongoing pressure for hospitals to use the lesser-paid nurses to do increasingly sophisticated tasks rather than by the highly paid doctors. The result has been what we see today, in which advanced practice nurses are doing much of what was formerly the practice of medicine and are continuing to take over their turf. All of this is thanks to financial incentives, which the caring approach vilifies.

I've just painted a picture of nurses working for money and benefitting from some business processes of hospitals. This is also what has created the untenable position of nurses being overworked and lacking the authority to make the job tenable. Employers will continue to dump more and more responsibility on any worker that accepts it until problems arise for that employer. Nurses are taking on the responsibility but hiding the negative consequences. Our sense of caring is often being used against us, in which a truly caring nurse would have worked harder to not make that error, and if she concerned about the patients she would not have called in sick.

The need to establish that significant personal bond with a patient is unnecessary for nurses in general and next to impossible in many cases. People come to us for a vast number of reasons, some of which fit the model of legitimate care, and many that do not. There is the drug seeking, malingering, or workers seeking documentation for that day they call in sick, regardless of whether they are ill or not. When a patient sees a nurse for a simple task, such as getting a vaccination, there is not much of a relationship at all. The vast majority of the work done by nurses consists of simple transactions.

Even in the acute care environment, substantial nurse/patient relationships are rare. When you look at the history of critical care nursing, patients are placed in departments or even hospitals, based on medical priorities, not relationships with any particular staff.[18] Scheduling of nurses is often chaotic, and matching nurses with individual patients to maintain an ongoing pairing rarely happens. If that pairing does happen, it has more to do with the fact that that nurse is familiar with the patient's care program than any relational reasons. EDs may have the frequent flyers, but the visits are brief and there is usually not one nurse seeing the same patient. In the ICU, there is the best chance of such a relationship occurring when there are long stays. Of course, if the patient is unconscious, there is not much of that relationship going on. It's also worth remembering that nurses are not the only ones at the bedside. The doctors and other providers are also there. One common theme of in-hospital stays is the large number of people coming into the patient's room, waking them up, invading their privacy, and so on. Even if there was a hope for a nurse to establish a relationship with a patient, there is a competition for the patient's time and attention against all the other providers.

The patient does not choose the RN, and even if a patient requests a specific nurse, such accommodations are infrequent. RNs do not stay in one place for long. Even if she is working in the same hospital, she may move to different departments, and very few stay at the same hospital for many years. If one sees a nurse and patient working together for extended periods of time, is this relationship any different from other professions? People get very attached to their housekeeper, or the waiter in their favorite restaurant. It is not clear that the medical services warrant a special category.

45

Imagine the ideal situation in which a nurse does have a substantial relationship with her patients. They know each other well and the nurse sincerely wants what is best for each and every one of her patients. Would that generate the model caring relationship? There is still another issue, that the nurse is not representing herself. She is representing her department, the hospital, and her profession. She is an employee and that patient has a relationship with the hospital, not with the nurse. State boards of nursing have repeatedly and consistently stated that nurses are to maintain a professional relationship with patients. In one case, a nurse employed in a mental health facility was disciplined for renting a spare room in her house to a person who had in the past been a patient at that mental health facility. The board based its decision on the assumption that, given the ex-patient's diagnosis, he was likely to be hospitalized at some point in his life, and his housemate would then be in a conflict of interest.

Also consider the effect a personal relationship has on one's decision-making. Clinical decision-making requires one to make rational choices under stressful conditions (see the chapter on smarts). If the nurse has an emotional attachment to a patient, it usually leads to worse decisions, not better ones. A key part of bad decisions comes from being emotionally and/or personally vested in the outcome.

One last concern of the nurse who develops a substantial relationship with a patient has to do with compatibility. You assume that an increasingly close bond between nurse and patient will always be a positive thing. If the nurse gets to know the patient more, why assume that would create a positive relationship? Maybe the nurse would actually grow to dislike the person more rather than feel that storied emotional bond, and that would not be good for the patient's care, either. Increased contact could produce conflict instead of cooperation.[19]

Consider the cases of Stuart, a patient with an artificial heart valve from when he got an infection at the age of 21. He takes warfarin, which nurses know to be a very problematic drug. It interacts with everything, and thus the need for frequent trips to the lab to watch his clotting factors. He was in South Africa on a vacation when he got sick and ended up in the hospital. At first, they put him in a hospital for blacks, but then soon transferred him to one for whites since this was the era of apartheid. He does not remember any of the nurses that cared for him.

Stuart is now in his 50s and has been in the hospital a few times.

Once he was put on a medication for gout, and that was enough to interact with the warfarin and cause a bleed, landing him in the hospital for a few days. I asked him about the care. One thing that he found annoying was the chaplain, who would come by every morning, asking if he wanted to talk to anyone about spiritual care. No, he did not. Stuart felt like a captive audience for the spiritual services folks. When I asked him about the care, he said it was excellent, but could not remember the name of any nurse. The same doctor was assigned to him for these few days, and that was the only person he could remember.

Nurses came and went. I'm thinking they were all caring in a professional way. If any of them disliked Stuart for any reason, it was not apparent. He is gay, and his husband was there every day. I know for a fact that some nurses do not like gays. A couple of my fellow nurses have confided in me that they don't think homosexuality is normal or acceptable, but they keep their opinions to themselves. It is not the concern for the patient that keeps them silent, said my two confidants, but simply that they want to keep their job. Statistically speaking, it is almost certain that some of Stuart's nurses had a personal issue with this.

The nursing profession is filled with people from all walks of life. There is a diversity of cultures and backgrounds that goes unseen because the role of a nurse forces us to conform. Working in a hospital means adjusting your values to meet the expectations of the patients and the employer. There are homophobes and racists in society, and some of them are nurses. The good news is that our professional values impel us to be better for the sake of the patient. On the flip side, a nurse, no matter how virtuous, often does not get credit for her work. No nurse would get particular credit for the services she provided to Stuart, on this hospitalization or any other. That is the reality we work with.

Caring and the interpersonal relationship matter more in some circumstances, and less in others. When does caring most matter? First, when the patient has no friends or family and needs his psychosocial needs met. Second, when there is a lot at stake, not when the patient is there for a simple transaction. And finally, caring matters most when there is the ongoing relationship or the possibility of such. When are all three of these three conditions fulfilled? Rarely.

Should we be looking for ways to increase these windows of opportunity? We still need to be cautious of an unintended side effect, the risk that you are disempowering the patient and his family and friends or creating a conflict of interest. If the nurse is going to enter into the role of the patient's advocate or the coordinator of patient care, she needs to look at that patient's circle of family/friends and see who would be better at doing this. There is a good chance that the patient already has a personal advocate, and that person needs to be empowered, not replaced. Patients want medical care, and the evidence strongly suggests that the less time spent with any clinicians, the better. Eric Topol, a doctor dubbed a "Rock Star of Science" by *GQ* magazine, coaches people on how to take control of their healthcare, urging people to not let the medical professionals run the program.[20] That much is not controversial. The implication is that patients want health services, not a relationship. Patients are not writing books about how they want to spend more time with nurses or doctors.

The nurses often seem to not want a relationship with individual patients. One of the reasons often cited by nurses for not wanting to work in the ICU is that you see the same patient for 12 hours, day after day. If caring is a primary motivating factor for nurses, one would expect to see the highest job satisfaction among those nurses that have the highest patient contact. The more contact with patients, and the higher the acuity, the higher the job satisfaction scores one should see. Yet we see the exact opposite happening. A survey was done of nurses, and higher patient contact correlated with lower job satisfaction.[21] Those working in long-term care facilities and hospitals were much less satisfied than nurse educators. It may be that the pay in nursing homes is less, and that would explain the lower satisfaction scores there. But the pay in hospitals exceeds the pay in academia, yet the nurse educators had much higher satisfaction scores than those in hospitals. When viewed by job position, the relationship was even more pronounced. Staff nurses were the least satisfied, first-line managers were in the middle, and senior managers were the happiest. Even with all the stress and pressures associated with senior management, being further away from patients seems to correlate with higher job satisfaction.

Consider emotional boundaries, which are found in all relationships, from the most intimate, as with a spouse, to the most distant, as with a stranger. In cases of complete strangers meeting for the first time, there are boundaries associated with establishing some safe interaction between these two. Given the spectrum between spouses on one end and complete strangers on the other, where is the nurse/patient relationship? Actually, quite close to that of a stranger. Yet there is also that need to create a relationship in a very fast manner because there are patient needs to be met. That is one of the unique challenges of nursing. Are the boundaries based on professional distance, or should the nurse strive for something personal and intimate? We are faced with a contradiction, at one time being told to push for a personal and intimate relationship, yet at the same time respect boundaries that preserve the patient's privacy and autonomy.

If a nurse is supposed to provide all patients with love and tenderness, a great injustice is being done to the nurse's family, friends, and, well, loved ones. Imagine if a person says she loves you, and then goes on to say she has a genuine love for all people. The message is clear. The love for you is nothing particularly special.

One nurse, Karen, presented with this issue, thought of a scenario in which she could treat her patient like family. She described how she could treat a young girl with cancer just like her own children. Fair enough, I responded. She seemed like a very caring nurse, one that Nightingale could be proud of. Would she stay after her 12-hour shift and spend the night at bedside? Would she have countless sleepless nights wondering how her life would be when this girl dies? Is the nurse going to mortgage her house to pay for the medical bills? The case of the young girl with cancer is one of the more sympathetic examples she could have drawn up. What if the patient were a 50-year-old rich white male who came into the ED acting manipulative, belligerent, and threatening to sue the nurse? Would there have been any impulse – much less an attempt – to treat him like family?

Clearly, nurses do not treat patients anything close to family, and should not. Karen realized that her view of caring was selective, in which she applied it to one case, the dying child, and did not think of the other cases. We all have that tendency to compartmentalize, feeling a certain way in some cases, but then apply different standards to a similar case that does not fit out thinking.

As if feeling the right way and acting the right way was not enough, some nursing scholars, such as Watson, are saying nurses need to share their own stories and feelings with the patients.[22] Just how much of the nurse's personal life should be shared with a patient that is already coping with his own medical issues? Clearly none. Intimacy is a two-way

49

relationship, which means that if we are going to connect with the patient's most personal feelings, the nurse needs to share hers. However, that is not part of the deal when one takes on a job as a nurse. If the nurse is going to share intimacy with patients, it means the nurse is dumping her worries and concerns on the patients. Emotional labor, which we just discussed, refers to an entire area of the economy in which the worker adjusts her feelings in order to have a desired effect on others in the professional environment.[23] This includes entertainers, the hospitality industry, and anywhere you expect that service provider to have a given demeanor for your benefit. When you shop in a store, you do not want to hear about that salesman's problems. Emotional labor better describes nursing, in which the nurse changes her demeanor to meet the needs of the patient, and never the opposite.

Nurses have a professional commitment to treat all patients the same, but the daily reality of nursing dictates otherwise. Ideally, all patients get a certain level of care that is appropriate, but some are simply not going to get that "loving" care. If you have strong ethical standards, then those that violate social norms should elicit an emotional response. In other words, if a nurse is truly committed to the highest ideals of conduct for herself, it means making judgment calls on others. It is unrealistic to suggest that a nurse holding high moral standards for herself, which entails holding others accountable to make sure things are fair, would withhold judgment on patients who are violating those norms. Just because she does not show it does not mean the feelings are not there, yet the dominant caring literature states that your behaviors must be authentic.

Watson stated that caring can be quantified, leading to extensive efforts to measure the amount of caring, the quantity of caring provided, or the impact of caring. A common way of measuring it is to describe anything a nurse does as inherently caring. In other words, the simple acts of assessing a patient, administering medications, and so on, are caring acts. Nursing scholar Pauline Phillips thinks of this description of caring as a tautology.[24] When you describe nurse caring as doing any of those things that are part of a normal nursing job, then by definition she is caring. Instead of thinking of a caring person who is doing something extraordinary, any nurse is, by definition, caring. Those who have written about caring have cast a net so wide that it is no surprise something is getting caught. The range of behaviors, attitudes, or results that qualify as caring is so broad that measuring any will be an exercise in frustration.

I find few things notable, and concerning, about the movement toward quantification. First, a concept needs to be adequately specified before one tries to quantify it. Yet, the definitions of caring are far from clear. Another concern is that if something can be expected of everyone, can be learned and quantified, then it will eventually become part of the job requirements and enforced. Instead of being that authentic personality trait of a nurse, it can be one more task that is assigned and demanded. Consider Arizona's standard of unprofessional conduct. Caring is not part of it. As if that list were not long enough, and vague enough, imagine if they did try to add caring, or the lack thereof.

Gaming the system is standard procedure in any organization, and nursing is no exception. Whatever caring behaviors might be adopted by a hospital could be easily fulfilled in order to get the desired results from customer surveys. One could easily think of ways a nurse could make her caring score higher. Give the patient whatever he wants. Talk up the little things she is doing as if they were special, even if they are required anyway. Give that registry nurse the difficult patients that are going to drive down the caring scores. Any attempt to measure and manage human behaviors is challenging, but given the vague and contradictory ideas of caring, it will be simply a mess.

Patients were asked what they want from their nurse, and they consistently valued technical skills over caring. What patients valued was often, ignored. Nursing scholar Patricia Larson surveyed cancer patients in three hospitals in Northern California and found that whereas nurses focus on a psychosocial function, the patients focus on demonstrated professional competency.[25] The importance of this finding seems to have been overlooked. Patients have repeatedly stated that if they are forced to choose, they prefer technical expertise to the softer qualities of care. The results of Larson's study showed that the nurses' priorities were quite different from the patients' priorities. Instead of recognizing this, she goes on to say "by being fully aware of the importance patients attach to caring behaviors, nurse can then move on to the interactions which nurses find meaningful – touching, being receptive to patient's needs, and providing individualized care."[26] Larson seems to think the nurse is allowed to turn her job into that which she finds meaningful, and not what the patient wants. When this study was republished in a book of classic works on caring, the segments showing how patient priorities

51

were different from nurse priorities were mostly edited out.[27]

If there is an aspect of caring that is unique to nursing, it has yet to be described in a matter that is separate from doctors, or any other healthcare providers. Why do doctors not carry the title of caring? They face a far greater hurdle in their training and selection. To become a doctor is a much longer and more selective process. Doctors get credit for their caring work, but they do not seem to describe it in the same manner or make such emphatic use of the word. There has been an active debate among doctors as to the role of caring in their practice, given the pressures of time and money.[28] Nurses have declared that this profession has the special role as the patient's advocate, but that role is not uncontested. Lucian Leape, who has been called the godfather of patient safety, said, "As the patient's advocate, the physician must play the key role."[*29] Nursing has been distinguished from medicine in that we care for the entire person, and not just the illness. Again, doctors are also looking at the big picture of what a patient needs to be healthy and not just what illness brought him to the hospital. Georgetown Medical School's founding principle is *cura personalis*, a Latin term derived from a Jesuit concept of care for the whole person.

Caring and Gender Behavioral Differences

As I mentioned in the Preface, some of the material in this book is more experience-based. I would be remiss were I not to share some observations about caring in nursing that seem to be as much about gender behavioral differences than anything else.

Most of the research on the caring behaviors of nurses—it just so happens that most of the researchers are women—describes what the authors of those studies characterize as stereotypically feminine behaviors, but largely omit any discussion of gender differences in behavior. The result is that female behavior "norms" become the unstated baseline for whatever is discussed.

One thing I've found is that many nurses who have excluded me from their conversations just because I am male are very caring when it came to patients. It's an odd dichotomy that I've seen in every place I've worked as a nurse: one set of standards of conduct—*act caring*—toward

---

* The context was when there is an error and who among the treatment team must take responsibility.

patients; a totally different standard of conduct—*maybe caring, maybe not*—toward other nurses.

Any time I compare men and women, I have an almost overwhelming sense of not being able to generalize about gender roles. I don't feel comfortable saying men are more like this and women are more like that. Part of it, I suppose, is that I live in northern California, with its liberal, progressive culture in which sexism is probably far less tolerated (for want of a better word) than in some other parts of the country. Our region's large gay population also makes it difficult to generalize about gender roles. So, any discussion of gender differences is fraught with danger.

It's easy to say such and such behavior is only a stereotype, that not all women or all men do this or that, or to characterize a given behavior associated mostly with women as "good" and advocate that it ought to be men's behavior, too. Take communication, for instance, which is a key part of how those who study caring see it conveyed. Men and women are known to express themselves differently, but if that isn't taken into account, a description and study of "caring" behaviors can end up with the caring behaviors of male nurses not being seen as such.

The best I can do here is to share some of my experiences with the different ways women and men in our profession. In some examples from my own experience, you can see how this all gets mixed together, and how the different ways women and men behave plays out with respect to "caring."

Admittedly, I'm not drawing on anything "scientific" in making the gender differentiations in these examples, and they probably reveal as much about my own worldview than they do about anything else. While the nursing literature persists in making generalizations, my own hunch is that women cannot be viewed as inherently more caring than men. Of course, I've personally witnessed tremendous caring from female nurses. One time, I watched a nurse tend to an elderly woman who had been left alone in the Emergency Department without any family or friends around. The woman was not in any apparent distress, and I have no idea what medical problem brought her to the ED. She gave me the impression of someone alone in this world, stuck in a busy hospital surrounded by care providers who were supposed to treat her as a person. As the woman rested on a gurney in the hallway, the RN taking care of her spoon-fed her and spoke to her as if she was that nurse's own beloved grandmother.

That same caring nurse, by the way, was a major bully to me—but caring and bullying seem to be two sides of the same coin when it comes to many nurses.

A male nurse, to be sure, could have shown just as much caring for that elderly woman. And I don't recall a single instance in which I observed a male nurse acting brutish in the clinical environment. On the contrary, I have experienced men in nursing demonstrate tremendous "caring"—and always try to do that myself.

In any case, here are some more examples of differences between male and female nurses, beginning with dealing with kids as patients. Some of the examples are about little things; others are probably more noteworthy.

When I was still quite new in the pediatric emergency department, lots of things would happen I had never encountered in my prior position in a general, all-ages emergency department. One of them was blowing bubbles. Young children are often upset or downright scared when you're taking their vital signs. It's normal behavior for a kid in a medical setting. Blowing bubbles has a magical effect. It distracts kids, amuses them, and ultimately calms them down—which means you can get some realistic vitals.

Blowing bubbles for kids is not a feminine or masculine thing to do. In the pediatric emergency room, it is just a great idea that became a widespread practice among those who specialize in pediatrics.

Another time, though, something happened that I would never have imagined a guy doing. I was starting an IV on a child, who was getting upset. The other two nurses I was working with—both women— spontaneously burst out in song. They sang a nursery rhyme. There was nothing special about the particular song; they were just trying to calm the child down.

I had never before heard singing in a clinical setting before, and certainly not by the staff. I was the one starting the IV, and trying to focus on that. It was a little distracting having nurses singing inches away from my face, but the calming effect on the child was real. To me, that is classic female behavior—but maybe that's because I don't sing, ever. It's a good thing they weren't expecting me to join in.

Then there are other behaviors that I would describe as more likely to be done by men and that may not fit the stereotypical definition of caring. I include among these things that are distasteful or dangerous, but are the "right" thing to do at the moment. For instance, I once went out into the waiting room to see what the commotion was all about. There was a distraught father with a teenage girl who was sitting in a wheelchair he had put her in. She was screaming at nothing in particular, swinging her arms with fists clenched, and shaking her head wildly. It was clear she was having some sort of emotional issue.

The dad looked at me and explained that she has these outbursts and needs help. He also said she could lash out and warned me to be careful.

I used a control hold on her, putting her arm behind her back and thus restraining her. I had been trained on the hold and knew what I was doing; I would not suggest anyone try it without that training. I then put the girl on a gurney and rolled her into the emergency room, still restraining her.

A doctor walked up. He clearly did not like seeing the girl being held down, and demanded I let her go. I explained to him the situation, and the danger she posed. He shrugged off my concern.

"Let her go," he insisted.

At that moment, the girl snatched the pen from the doctor's breast pocket and began trying to stab him with it. I had expected something like that, grabbed her again before she could hit him, and put her back into a restraint. The doctor looked shocked. He acquiesced to having her restrained.

To some, that control hold may seem oppressive or mean. In that circumstance, I was doing the right thing. No one ever said a word about it, but I got the clear impression that some of the nurses did not approve. Obviously, though, as much as blowing bubbles and singing a song had helped with younger children, it was clear neither of those were going to work with that violent teenager.

From Caring to Professionalism

Nursing was founded on ideals that we can all be proud of, and it should come as no surprise that we are the most trusted profession. From these beginnings, I see a generational change in which we build on the works of Nightingale, Watson, and the many others who made it clear that we are not simply a profit-driven industry, but a group of dedicated workers that fill a vital role in people's lives. That has led us to the current situation in which we try to fulfill every demand that comes before us.

This is not workable. The point is not that we should not care, but that in order to help this patient, we need to set limits on ourselves. There is an alternative that has all the elements of caring without the unnecessary emotional baggage and unrealistic obligations. Caring can be conceptualized as professionalism, in which the nurse provides excellent healthcare to anyone, strangers and friends alike, with equal attention and diligence. Professionalism means keeping an arm's length distance and not taking things personally, which is almost always a better situation than subjecting oneself to the stress and burnout that will prevent the nurse from staying focused on her job.

By professionalism, I mean an approach to my job in which the patient's nursing needs will be addressed by me as much as possible given financial and organizational constraints. Some patient needs are not nursing needs, and most of the emotional and relational aspects of caring that we have just heard about do not fall into my job description. We have mental health professionals, case managers, and other specialists far better qualified to deal with these personal problems than a nurse. If a nurse wants to distinguish herself, do the best of what is within the nursing role, and coordinate with team members as they do their job.

We face pain, death, and conflict on a daily basis. No nurse should be reduced to tears for not having made the patient's life all better. To go back to my EMT instructor, the patient is having a crisis. It is his crisis, not ours. If you feel the need to become emotionally involved, your judgment is being colored and you will not be making the best choices for the patient.

There is a side benefit to the public perception of nursing as the caring profession. It gives us some advantage and protects the nurse. We have heard a lot about the need to document carefully, follow the rules, and act in the patient's best interest. Much of what we do cannot be easily documented, such as caring behaviors or critical thinking. We often need to do things that may be interpreted in different ways, such as how we touch a patient or whether we are protecting them from a fall versus pushing them around. We hear about cases against nurses that reach the court, yet when you look at the vast amount of nursing work done in our society—involving 3 million nurses and many millions of patients—litigation is actually quite rare. When a nurse does end up in that defendant's chair facing a jury of her peers, this is when the caring profession matters. When you come from the most trusted profession in our society, a jury is going to believe you unless they have compelling reasons to do otherwise. This is supposed to be the case in all court battles, in which the defendant is innocent until proven guilty, but we also know that juries are swayed by personalities and impressions made in the court room. And in this case, being a nurse is a strong plus. If a nurse comes across as overly sentimental, emotional, and violating patient boundaries, it is not clear how that will be help her when mistakes are made. However, the nurse as professional that cares about the patient but demonstrates restraint, discipline, and boundaries, may have a better outcome.

Nursing leaders also follow the ethical standards even when there is no direct patient care, and from what we have seen, caring does not translate well to the executive suite. Professionalism does. Hospitals need to make harsh choices, based on money and power, running the organization in a sustainable manner. If you are not willing to accept limits on caring as a bedside nurse, how would you do so as a supervisor? And from those supervisors come our managers and executives. The expectations of nurses at any level of the organization should not be any different.

Chapter 2 References
* Gorrell, *Heart and Soul.*
2 Donelan *et al.,* Public Perceptions of Nursing Careers."
3 Williams, "Literature Review."
4 Strickland, "Foreword."
5 Watson, *Assessing and Measuring Caring in Nursing and Health Sciences.*
6 Personal communication with the author.
7 Bradshaw, "Measuring Nursing Care and Compassion."
8 Hochschild, *The Managed Heart.*
9 Achen and Bartels, *Democracy for Realists.*
10 Graeber, *The Good Nurse.*
11 Rhodes *et al,* "Nursing at Its Best."
12 Spetz and Herrera, "Changes in Nursing Satisfaction in California."
13 Semega, "Median Household Incomes for States."
14 AFL-CIO, "Nursing: A Profile of the Profession."
15 Smith, "Florida Is Facing Another Nursing Shortage."
16 Kingma, Mireille, *Nurses on the Move;* Choy, *Empire of Care.*
17 See, for example, Weinberg, *Code Green.*

[18] Zalumas, *Caring in Crisis.*

[19] Norton, *et al.*, "Less Is Often More."

[20] Topol, *The Patient Will See You Now.*

[21] HRSA, "The Registered Nurse Population," chapter 3.

[22] Wolf *et al.*, "Dimensions of Nurse Caring."

[23] Hochschild, *The Managed Heart*; Smith, *The Emotional Labour of Nursing.*

[24] Phillips, "A Deconstruction of Caring."

[25] Kyle, "The Concept of Caring"; Larson, "Important Nurse Caring Behaviors …"

[26] Larson, *ibid.*

[27] Smith *et al.*, *Caring in Nursing Classics.*

[28] Rosenberg, *Our Present Complaint.*

[29] Leape, "Apology for Errors."

3
From Information to Smarts

Learning the role of nurse for me took place in three phases. In the first, as an EMT on an ambulance, the world of healthcare was laid before me like never before. I'm rather healthy and have not spent much time in hospitals. They were foreboding and smelly places, better to be avoided. Now in my next career, they were exciting and offered a chance for employment. I was doing a fly-along with Stanford Hospital's Life Flight, the medical helicopter service. For one day, they allowed me to wear their flight suit and hang out in their office until there was a call. Another medivac helicopter arrived that morning, and we assisted. The doors opened and the insides were covered in blood. A 21-year-old guy enrolled in a work training program in the Santa Cruz area had his legs crushed in a machine called, ironically, The Crusher. One leg was completely detached, the other half detached. As we rolled him across the roof to the elevator, down to the first floor, and to the ED, he looked at a nurse pushing the gurney and asked, "Is my leg okay?." She just looked at him and said, "No, it looks like you may have lost one of them."

Her composure was amazing. I so wanted to be a nurse like that.

Then we entered the ED's trauma room. Instead of a smooth and organized process, I saw chaos and confusion. There were about 25 people in the room, some doing a clearly recognized task, others seemingly just there. One young man asked me where a certain piece of equipment could be found. I'm not familiar with this ED, I told him. He seemed confused, since I was wearing the flight suit. Another nurse at the patient's side was doing a head to toe assessment. The patient was naked with a gown tossed over his mid-section. She leaned over to look him in the eye and said, "I need to see your penis. Is that OK?" He just looked at her with a blank stare, and she just went ahead with her assessment of the pelvic area.

After what seemed like forever, an older white man—the caricature of a senior doctor—said loudly, "You need to wrap this up!" He then began counting down, "Ten, nine, eight…" Everyone scrambled, and as he got to one, the other flight nurse and I pushed the gurney out of the ED and upstairs to the surgical area. There, things were entirely different. I recall quiet and calm, and everyone's movements were precise and smooth. There was a line on the floor, at which point their nurse took over the patient and the gurney. My job was done.

My lesson from all this was that nurses work in stressful, high stakes environment, but it cannot be assumed that everyone knows their role. It is up to the nurse to accomplish as much as possible depending on the environment in which she works.

The second phase of my education played out in the first day and weeks of nursing school. Erin, my classmate, was an Asian man in his late 40s with a PhD in acupuncture. He was excited to make a career shift to nursing. I would say it was a shift and not a change because, in his mind, acupuncture and nursing were just two ways to provide care to a patient. At this point I had already spent a large amount of time in the ambulance and over a year as an ED tech. All the nurses told me was that nursing school does not teach you much. Time spent in a hospital with patients is where you learn. Being the cynic, I told Erin we were not going to learn much in this program. We were there to get two magic letters, an R and an N. It was an accelerated, one-year BSN program at a private school, so it was a little pricey. He thought I was being a downer.

That first couple of weeks, we were taught nursing theories and nursing diagnoses; the hands-on portion was how to wash our hands. Nursing diagnoses were being taught as a way for our profession to assert itself. Doctors made medical diagnoses, and nurses could make nursing diagnoses. We could diagnose a patient with "risk for loneliness" or "disturbed energy field." This seemed bizarre to me. My classmates dutifully took notes and believed most of what they were being told. I went back to my weekend job in the ED and asked the nurses about nursing diagnoses. They uniformly agreed that these "diagnoses" were a joke. Unfortunately, joke or not, we were being told a nursing diagnosis was required in our charting.

My lesson from nursing school was that the training of a nurse is long, expensive, and cannot be counted upon to prepare a nurse to work in a hospital. We graduated and most of us were hired in hospitals, but there was this major disconnect between what was being taught and what we needed to get and keep that first job.

The third phase was my new nurse program in the ED. I already mentioned some of my experiences there. The lessons learned after a year in the ED were what I found useful. Anticipate what the doctors and nurses want and need. Be diplomatic to the patient's family members. Most importantly, work hard and don't sit at the nursing station. The experienced nurses can sit there. It does not look good when a new nurse is spending time sitting at the nursing station.

These three phases taught me that nursing is a profession and not just a trade, and that nurses are knowledge professionals. Nurses have moved from the relatively unskilled handmaidens of doctors to professional healthcare clinicians, while the volume and breadth of knowledge a nurse needs to have mastered has grown many-fold. I found the term we used in school, nursing knowledge, did not capture what was going on here. For the nurse, possessing knowledge was not enough. It is what she does with it that matters. Smarts is not a common term used in nursing, and I use it here to refer to something much broader than nursing knowledge.

Understanding the role of smarts is important because the profession requires highly skilled nurses, yet it has proven a little tricky to describe what exactly is meant by that word *skilled*. There is a large volume of information that must be held by the nurse, which means we need to be judicious in what is important, what is optional, and what is a lesser priority. When a nurse is deemed unskilled or, worse yet, incompetent, we need to be very clear about what is lacking. Nursing schools struggle to understand what information needs to be covered in the program, how to teach it, and how to test for it. The educational level of nurses has been shown to improve patient outcomes.[1] Nursing boards judge applicants to decide who gets a license and who does not. Overall, nursing smarts is critically important to this profession and society's health status. If we fail to require a sufficient level of smarts in our nurses, we end up with an unsafe practice. It is not just the amount of knowledge that matters but also the specific things that nurses need to know.

Knowledge is also expressed in groups and organizations, and the hospital may help or hinder the process. Teamwork is mostly a matter of sharing knowledge and information. Nurses work with other nurses and a dizzying array of doctors, specialists, administrative staff—not to mention patients and their families. A nurse can use the team to coast along and not carry her own weight or support the team for which she may or may not get credit.

What is Smarts?

We hear a lot of different terms such as *nursing knowledge*, *critical thinking*, *intuition*, and so on. But what exactly is *smarts*? I define it as all the things a nurse needs to understand and demonstrate, with an appropriate attitude that allows the nurse as an individual to perform her duties and, as a group, for nursing to develop as a profession.

Sherry, the ED nurse I introduced earlier, was one of the best nurses I have ever worked with. She had been at Marin General Hospital's ED for several years and was one of the key players in that department, and the entire hospital. When she took me on as a preceptor, she navigated the noise and confusion to focus on what mattered most at any one time.

A middle aged Hispanic man walked up to the ambulance door, his face covered in blood, and his lips slashed wide open. He was drunk and had fallen down some stairs. Sherry walked him to the trauma bay, while pointing to a doctor to indicate who was needed at bedside. It was soon apparent a translator was needed, and Sherry asked for the one person she knew to be in the area that was a Spanish speaker. While I started the IV, Sherry was assembling the team of specialists that needed to be there, even before the doctor was done with his initial head to toe assessment. The other patients assigned to her could wait, but not too long. She directed me to check in on the other patient with a IV infusion in case there was a reaction to the medication, and let the other patient, who did not have an urgent issue, to please be understanding while we deal with this emergency.

Sherry demonstrated the ability to perform skills, including simple tasks and complex critical thinking, in a variety of conditions—including this high stress clinical setting. When things were quiet, she could also give me a mini-lesson on nursing skills or things I would need to do to get through my nursing program. A major theme in acute care nursing is that working under stressful conditions affects judgment. Having information available in a relaxed environment is not the same as using it in an emergency.

Sherry's skill here is not something that could be taken for granted. Another nurse in that same unit got upset one day when there were no crutches in the supply room, and he refused to answer questions for the next hour, even when things had quieted down. Communications is intimately tied to smarts. If you cannot act on a problem because you cannot communicate about it clearly, it does not matter what knowledge you may have. Simply having information is irrelevant if it cannot be used in the clinical environment. The point was made in the discussion of caring that we need to distinguish between behaviors and the thoughts or feelings that may be driving the behaviors. With smarts, the same thing applies. Nurses need to demonstrate knowledge of a wide variety of things, but the important part is to demonstrate it.

Challenges

If Sherry's example was the standard, then nursing would be in a great position. The average nurse struggles to employ her smarts in stressful condition, making good decisions that make everyone happy. We are overloaded with information and face multiple hurdles in employing the right information in the right context. To be reasonable, if you want more of one thing, you should allow less of something else. Sherry succeeded by filtering out what is not important so she can make good decisions in those areas that mattered most at that moment. Still, she is the exception. Few nurses could do as good a job as she did.

My concern here is that we need to look at the average nurse, not just the exceptional ones. Our current system seems to use the best nurses as exemplars and say, if she can do it, why can't you? The answer to his has been *Just Culture* (the focus of a later chapter). My point here is to show how nurses are being called upon to know more than one can reasonably be expected to know, employ that information in a high stress environment, and not make mistakes. A reasonable person would say if you want more of one thing, you need to have less of something else. If you want me to learn the newest clinical science and technology, then I may not have the time or attention to also read the newest hospital policies. That is not what is happening. Our hospitals, and the outside forces behind them, are dumping more information demands on nurses.

We as a society have done a poor job of identifying what tradeoffs can be made if you want more of something. Sherry's hospital introduced a new information system, which was supposed to reduce errors and make his job easier. Instead, it was up to her and the other nurses to fix the bugs in the system while they were still providing patient care. To be fair, there was a grace period in which everyone was learning the system. But after a couple months, the workload did not change. What did change was that her work was now being recorded in minute detail, in real time. Errors were expected to go down. Instead of saving Sherry any effort, she was now faced with increased expectations and lower tolerance for mistakes.

Atul Gawande, a doctor who writes for *The New Yorker*, notes that ignorance is when we do not have the knowledge, but ineptitude is when we have the knowledge but do not apply it correctly.[2] We are seeing a major shift from historical lack of knowledge to the present era in which we are struggling with information overload, which gets in the way of what Gawande calls our *eptitude*. A major part of Sherry's work was to research the patient's history. Her decisions depended heavily on the patient's prior history, what treatments he has received, and how he responded to those interventions. I was surprised how difficult it could be to get a history. Some hospital systems like the Veterans Administration and Kaiser Permanente have excellent information systems that capture vast amounts of data. In other hospitals, patient's come in with little or no documentation, and sometimes, in a clinic or in the ED, we are not even sure who this person really is. As Sherry's hospital introduced the new information system, she was expected to know more and more of the patient's history, even when it was hidden in the system. When something bad happened and an audit was done, it is easy to find patient information in the system that was not apparent to Sherry at that crucial moment. Yet it was somewhere in the records, and she was expected to find it. Again, the demands made of her kept going up, even when the hospital was introducing changes that were supposed to lessen the load.

The stress nurses face comes from working in life or death environments where a mistake can have fatal consequences. But the nature of stress is not always well understood. Those who already work as a nurse have already mastered that challenge, more or less. What of all those people that could have been a nurse but where turned away from the profession? I often hear people say, "I would have liked to be a nurse, but…" and that sentence ends with something about body fluids, needles, or the human body. This reminds me that nurses are not typical. Most people have an ick factor, in which they cannot deal with those things that are gross or dirty. Such a person may have all the intelligence and information of a nurse, but smarts requires her to overcome the distractions to get the job done. Even for those of us that are working as nurses, many feel the stress of working on human bodies, particularly when things get messy.

Todd was a nursing student who volunteered at an ED where I was working. He was determined to make himself a great nurse. One afternoon in the trauma room, I had a patient with excruciating pain in his belly. The doctor grabbed the ultrasound and saw an aortic aneurism that could burst at any moment. This patient's life was in the balance. The hospital called for a helicopter because we did not have the surgical services he needed. In those few minutes, it was my job to get two large bore IVs in. What also needed to happen was for the patient's clothes to be cut off. Todd jumped to it without hesitation. That is when we noticed the bowel movement. One reaction the patient had to his pain was to release his bowels, and it was a large, loose pile of poo smeared all over his underwear and beyond. The smell was quite profound. As I was busy getting in the IVs, I looked around, and Todd was nowhere to be seen. It was up to me to get the patient cleaned up. If he's going to surgery, having feces smeared all over is not going to work.

Todd was in the hallway, with a sheepish look. He apologized forcefully, saying he was going to vomit from the smell of the feces. Was I upset that he abandoned me? Yes and no. I would not use the word "abandon" in this case, but this was a good lesson for him. Sometimes, even clinicians get nauseous from the patient, even to the point of vomiting. If that happens, you go to the bin, get rid of your lunch, and get back to work. The patient is not concerned about seeing you sick so much as he was concerned about dying. It's OK for a nurse to be human. But you still need to do the job. To this day, I still remember the smell of that particular patient, and how the stress made it all the more challenging to make the right clinical decisions at that moment. This is something other nurses seem to have internalized. I notice it because for me nursing is a second career. As for Todd, he had smarts all along, which in this case meant the ability to learn from the experience.

In the busy clinical environment, nurses often make decisions that need a doctor's order—the best example being medications. Yet it has been standard practice for doctors to cover the nurse after the medication was given. This was being done on a routine basis in Sherry's ED by herself and most of the other nurses. Doctors simply did not have time in an emergency to enter the orders. In some cases, the doctor was busy with an emergency while Sherry handles the other patients, which included giving some medications that required an order. With the old paper documentation, it was easy to make things look appropriate even when this covering was being done. Under the new, electronic system, they know when Sherry is accessing the medication and if there was an order at that time. Her scope of authority was now being reduced just at the time when the demands made of her were increasing.

It is not just the hospitals that are upping the demands. There are many nurses arguing for more emphasis on whatever issues interest them. For example, some are calling for more training on cultural competence and others want more spiritual care. Erin, my classmate from nursing school, went on to work in a local hospital's med-surg unit. He told me of his planned proposal to management that what his patients needed was acupuncture. He thought acupuncture would be a useful addition to the other medical interventions performed. Another nurse was asking management for more opportunities to provide spiritual care to the patients. Instead of making the broader argument that we were simply too busy, these nurses were diplomatically told their ideas were nice and would be considered. Then they were ignored. Which I consider a good thing.

Part of Sherry's challenge is to keep up with the information load. The other part was that her performance was being assessed based on the unreasonable assumption that what was being demanded of her was reasonable. Like many nurses, she would occasionally complain of the workload, but nothing much would happen. There was never any major review by the hospital of all the demand parts of his or any other nurse's job position. Instead, she was doing what countless other nurses were doing. Those things that were not according to policy were covered up, and errors did not get reported. It was simply impossible for her, one of the best nurses, to meet all the demands made of her. For other nurses that were not as strong as her, the situation was dire. It was a game of setting up the work environment to avoid accountability in the first place, and work with other nurses that supported you. In this environment, a nurse, as a matter of career survival, demonstrates smarts by breaking some rules while maintaining patient safety.

Sherry's official job description offered a good example of what is wrong with this system. She, like most nurses, was required to sign a document acknowledging her job description and expectations. Hers looked essentially the same as the others I have seem from other hospitals. It is vague, including "Initiating personal contact" and "Ability to influence people." One thing her job description did not have, but I see on many others, was an ending statement such as "Any other task or duties deemed necessary." In other words, the hospital is telling Sherry her job duties are as broad as one could possible describe without any real limits.

The nursing profession is not getting better in matching experience and skills with job demands. If anything, it may be getting worse. Cost-cutting measures have included things like moving nurses between departments and more use of registry nurses. One of the greatest challenges to the cognitive skills of a nurse is to be put into a new department or a new facility, but this practice is becoming more common. Sherry knew everything about her department, and almost everything about the hospital. She could tell you which nurses would answer the phone in the ICU depending on the time and day, and how they would respond to getting a new patient just before shift change. She knew that if you needed supplies from the central warehouse, some would always be available and some would not. Much of nursing has nothing to do with nursing. It has all to do with being in your job long enough to figure out the flow of things.

Bana was a registry nurse who would often get assigned to this ED, and she stood out for her lack of orientation. No matter how good a nurse she was, and she had a wealth of experience, it did not matter when she didn't know where to find things or who to call for consults, room assignments, and so on. Yet the level of performance required of her was essentially the same. Registry nurses, RNs hired from agencies to work as temporary contractors, doing the same work as the other RNs, are becoming increasingly common as hospitals try to cut corners. They can claim that the standards are the same, but that is a little misleading. Sherry's job demand increases as she is expected to orient the registry nurses that appear on a regular basis. She does not get any particular credit for this extra work.

Another challenge to our cognitive skills is that we work in an environment that is highly intolerant of mistakes. Other industries can do things that we cannot. Google went from nothing to a market value of $400 billion dollars for a number of well-recognized managerial practices. Instead of seeking a 10 percent improvement, they were looking for a 10x (as in 10 times) improvement. Success was mostly due to some of their business practices. They sought to "fail fast." Instead of avoiding failure, they sought to make mistakes early and fast, learn from them, and move on. Instead of a *knowing* culture, they preferred *learning*. They also valued data over experience, intuition, or hierarchy.[3]

But Google's staff does not make the life or death decisions that every acute care nurse must face. We do not have the luxury of failing in any of our operations, though some leaders in our profession claim otherwise. The president of the American Association of Critical Care Nurses, for instance, said in a 2013 editorial that failure is okay and we should accept it and learn from it.[4] It is hard to imagine any significant example in which a nurse in acute care can fail where it does not jeopardize patient care directly or indirectly. The end result is both good and bad. The good news is that we are not expected to come up with revolutionary ideas that are going to change the operations of any department or hospital. You are free to ignore the management hype. In some other industries, your job will depend on coming up with brilliant ideas of change. Not so in nursing. The bad news is that we must stay above the tsunami of information hitting us every day in the clinical setting, and not make any major mistakes.

Defining Nurse Competence

I've painted a picture in which nurses are overwhelmed with the workload, the knowledge load, and the stressful environment in which they need to demonstrate their nursing skills. That leads to the question about competence. How do we determine whether a nurse is competent? I could not find clear and consistent definitions or even guidelines on what to look for. There has been a tug of war between the nursing schools, which want nurses that are adaptive, contemplative, and with some theory, and the hospitals, which want a workforce available with minimal cost and delay.

One name that comes up a lot is Patricia Benner, nursing scholar and author of one of the most famous books in our profession, *From Novice to Expert*. She took a practical and specific approach and placed the "competent" nurse in the middle of her continuum of nurse education, between advanced beginner and "proficient." The competent nurse is able to make plans and anticipate actions but lacks speed and flexibility.[5]

We start our careers by getting an RN license, which I find a little odd. All of this talk about the theory and measurement of our practice, and all of the testing done in nursing school, comes down to one license. Either you have it or you don't. When I worked as an ED tech, the nurses told me not to worry about grades, because nobody cares much about them. It is not looked upon kindly if you brag about your GPA to nurses. What nurses want to know if, can you do the job in a clinical environment? Can you start an IV? Can you see when a patient is in trouble? Sure enough, I graduated from nursing school with the lowest GPA in the class (that was a passing grade, of course), and was the first one hired. Benner's idea of novices turning into experts was all about the result, but not about what it takes to become that expert.

As I approached the end of my nursing program, it was time to get that first job. My ideal choice was the hospital right across the bridge from where I lived—part of a major hospital system and offering a busy ED. Having worked in another hospital as a tech, I was in the system. I showed up at the ED triage desk and asked to see the ED manager. Within minutes, I was meeting with one of the managers, who asked me to come back in a couple hours to interview. By chance, they were interviewing that day. The nurse interviewing me gave me three scenarios. This should all be familiar to every nurse. One patient was pale, cool, diaphoretic, complaining of chest pain. The next patient was pink, warm, and dry, with blood in his IV that had been saline locked. The third patient was complaining of nausea, but vital signs were normal. Which patient would I address first, and why? After all those months of training and testing, it all came down to that one question about triage. That was how this hospital deemed me competent.

As a nurse moves along her career, measuring competence does not seem to get much more sophisticated. I was able to move from that first job to the next simply by virtue of the fact that I had managed to pass the new RN program. As best I can tell, that was the only piece of information, and an interview with the same triage question, by which the next hospital picked me. The main thing that seems to get added to this process is the use of references. Employers depend heavily on references, particularly from your current job. Reputation matters, but it is filtered through that use of references. In other words, the main way we determine the competence of a nurse is that person we know something about, like a trusted fellow worker, who also knows the nurse applying for a job.

Another way to define competence is simply the lack of incompetence.[6] This has some merit, in that a nurse is far more likely to run into problems for making mistakes than for demonstrating some lesser standard of competence. Also, we tend to recognize acts of incompetence much more easily than the opposite. The problem is that once you make a mistake, your fellow workers can either dismiss it, or make it into a major issue. This is where bullying comes into play, which I will discuss later. If a nurse does not like you, she can simply wait for a mistake, make a complaint, and that is very likely to end up with some paper trail that makes your career move a lot more problematic.

That almost happened to one nurse who, by luck, was not in a job search at the time of her incident. Cynthia is a manager in a major middle-American town at one of their premier hospitals. She was in the midst of a highly contentious divorce, which as anyone who has gone through that knows, means that everything in your life can become an issue. She abides by the law more than most, but as I've said repeatedly, the nursing system is stacked against us in some key ways. We are going to break some rules no matter how honest or strict we try to be. She had some Tylenol with codeine in her house from a prior injury. Think of how many households in this country have a jar of narcotics in the cupboards because someone had had a medical procedure and did not need all those painkillers. Her friend down the street was in pain, and Cynthia, being a competent nurse, knew a couple of these pills would tide the friend over. She gave the friend a couple narcotic pills, which is a crime. When you get a prescription for a narcotic, only you can use it. Not only was she diverting a controlled substance, but she was also prescribing a medication, sort of, and dispensing. A few different crimes going on here. Still, I cannot imagine what kind of person would tell a close friend that they needed to either suffer the pain or go to the ED that night, incurring hundreds of dollars in copay, rather than give him a couple pills.

Now back to the divorce. The soon to be ex-husband knew of this, and you can see where this could have played out. He threatened to report her to the state nursing boards. The accusation involved narcotics, so I am confident it would have gone forward to investigations. I am not so confident honesty would have served her well in this case. If she admitted to the whole thing, the board would possibly discipline her. If she simply kept quiet and denied everything, I believe the case would have been dismissed for lack of evidence. Smarts in this example was demonstrated by discretely taking care of her friend's pain management without getting caught for diverting a narcotic.

What does this have to do with competence? It has everything to do with the way we treat nursing competence as a minimal standard. Cynthia's current job was never at risk because of their *Just Culture* policy. However, if she were making a job change, they would have asked her if she is under investigation, and she would have had to say yes. No matter that the case would ultimately be thrown out. The point here is that we either judge nurse competence by absolute rock bottom standards such as being licensed and no disciplinary actions, or by reputation. The nursing profession is trying to get credit for being skilled professionals, yet we often see our performance judged by the simplest of standards.

Assessing Nurses

The situation just described applies mostly to new nurses or when you are changing jobs. A different scenario plays out when the nurse needs to justify her actions in the course of her daily duties. The easiest way to stay out of trouble, we are told, is to follow the rules. Know the hospital's policies and procedures, and that will keep me out of trouble. I've already made the point that there are too many rules to follow, and real-world events are not so clear-cut. Nurses often need to explain their actions on day-to-day events that may appear to violate policies. This happens on a regular basis in every department I have every worked in. Instead of justifying herself as a nurse, she needs to justify a specific decision or action. If you can justify your actions, you can claim to be a safe nurse. However, consider all the different sources of guidance a nurse may use:

- Research
- Peer reviewed journals
- Professional journals
- What was taught in nursing school
- What the preceptors said
- Hospital policy/protocol
- Other hospital policy/protocol
- Common practice in the department
- What your supervisor said
- What the doctor said

In my role as a BLS instructor, I get to ask my students what they are doing in their facility. It turns out there has been a shift in how we use intra-osseus (IO) needles. In the past, the standard route was through the tibeal tuberosity. In other words, you put the IO in the bone just below the knee. Most trauma hospitals in my area are putting the IOs in the humeral head. Both sites are considered appropriate by the IO manufacturers, and I have not heard anything that compels one to use one location or the other. But the clinicians in the major EDs seem to have gravitated to the humeral site.

Donna, who works in a small community hospital, told her co-workers that they should be doing the same. If the major trauma EDs are using the humerus for IO insertions, why not them? Managers ignored her. There was even a poster on the wall of the ED from the IO manufacturer showing the acceptable insertion sites, which of course included the humerus. She was told to stick to policy. But wait: There is no policy! She told me how her managers reacted, asking if there was any research that could sway their opinion. I told her the sad fact that if a nursing manager is not willing to believe a poster from the manufacturer staring her in the face, no number of scholarly articles is going to make a difference. Stick to what the manager wants.

Donna's is not an isolated case. Nurse managers are also being overwhelmed by the overload of information, and they too are trying to make their jobs manageable. Instead of the additional information pushing our profession forward, I am seeing cases like this where it is keeping us from moving forward.

Solutions: Experience, Intuition, and Heuristics

Sherry has figured out how to make her job workable in the ED, as had Cynthia as a nursing manager. The stresses and struggles I have described are obviously not impossible to overcome since we usually get through the day and keep our job and license. There are a couple major things that Sherry and Cynthia count on to meet the information needs of their jobs. The main one is experience, that quality of nurses that takes a central role in how we are assessed and what qualifies a person for a given role. Sherry and Cynthia both have many years of nursing experience behind them, all of which was in hospitals and in the higher acuity departments. Sherry worked in an inner city hospital's ICU for the first 8 years of her career before moving to this suburban hospital ED. Cynthia has always worked in the same hospital in various in-patient departments.

Much of what is attributed to experience is not actually clinical knowledge. Nursing school taught me generic aspects of patient care, but organizational issues make all the difference in the real world. My success depends on knowing how the clinical environment works. Where do I find the on-call doctor? How do you call a trauma code? Where do blood samples go? Even documentation is more about knowing where to click for past lab results and what forms to fill out. A large percentage of my mental energy goes to things that have nothing to do with nursing. Major hospital incidents occur in July and August, when new cohorts of clinicians start working.[7] If there is a bump in these months that goes away in the fall, that is not experience as we know it. These doctors do not become experienced clinicians in a few months. Their familiarity with the workflow and the organization is at least as important, if not more so, than clinical skills.

The human brain has a lot of tricks to help us survive, and some of those tricks deal with how we process information and discern what is important. For example, emotions have been recognized as a form of intelligence, and can be used to help us make decisions, even in times of stress. The emotional brain buys time to give the rational brain a chance to process,[8] but we cannot always count on these mental processes for having the desired outcomes. Daniel Kahneman, a Nobel Prize winner in economics, and his partner Amos Tversky, showed how these tricks of mental processing can also go wrong.[9] Heuristics, they noticed, are used as mental tools to apply simple rules that help us make sense of complex situations. The problem is, sometimes they give us the wrong answer. If your subconscious is making decisions based on rules that you are not aware that you even have, it is very hard to check yourself.

For example, when a patient arrives into the ED and appears to be in stress, what is the sequence of events that Sherry needs to make happen? BLS is an algorithm when someone seems to be unresponsive. It can also be viewed as a heuristic, a simple way to make the best decision when she is bombarded with information and tasks. She checks for responsiveness while looking for breathing effort. If the patient is not responsive, she calls for help, then starts CPR. I find it a little odd that we are so comfortable with CPR, given the damage that it does. Chest compressions done well are likely to break ribs and cause internal bleeding. In fact, when I have a frail older person arrive in the ED and the medics tell me CPR was done on this patient in the field, I expect to see broken ribs. If the patient does not have broken ribs, it tells me the CPR may not have been done very well. Yet nurses are perfectly comfortable with this drastic action that could cause a lot of harm. This is because we have learned that CPR is the best thing to do when you have an unresponsive patient and cannot feel a pulse.

While a heuristic, BLS is also a standardized practice, a policy, and something we all need to be certified in to keep our jobs. Many heuristics are informal and personal. They can be considered your own way of making a decision that works for you. Sherry shared with me her smarts by teaching me one of her ways to manage her job. When a patient comes into the ED, what is needed to get this person back out the door so he can go home or be admitted to the appropriate hospital department. This is mostly an ED thing, but other departments use it to varying degrees. The ED is not where we solve all the problems. It is for emergencies. Some people think their ingrown toenail is an emergency. It is not. There are a few things that need to happen before a critically ill patient can be sent up to the ICU. The blood pressure needs to be something adequate. No active CPR. Not in an unstable rhythm. The standards vary depending on the hospital and what the ICU nurses consider acceptable. But Sherry's concern is to get that critically ill patient just stable enough to make it ICU's patient, and no longer hers. I would consider this practice a heuristic because it involves taking what could be a highly complex decision and making it simple and workable. Sherry is not trying to solve all of his patient's problems. When things get busy, she needs to just solve the emergency, and let others take over for the long-term care.

Hospitals try to create labor saving processes and ways to help us simplify our jobs. In other words, our employers are actively trying to create heuristics as a management technique. Some of these, like BLS, work well. Others do not. Any management process has costs and benefits. We nurses are being overwhelmed with information, which often comes from these misguided attempts to make our job easier. How many times have you heard this new process or the new form that needs to be filled out "will only take a few seconds"? Yes, but I would need to remember to fill out that form in the first place, and those seconds add up. For example, my ED sometimes has a stroke code. I am supposed to recall all of the things that need to be done to prepare a cardiac patient for a catheter lab that needs to be done within 90 minutes. Yet when we looked at how well that supposedly labor- and life-saving process works, it only happens about half the time, even though this is a relatively standard drill.[10]

Gawande, who developed the concept of *eptitude*, is also a big advocate of checklists. He shows how, in some cases, following a checklist can keep clinicians from making errors. Sure, checklists can make a big improvement in safety in some specific and isolated cases, but the reality of what nurses do on a constant basis in the fast-paced clinical environment does not fit any checklist. Sherry had a checklist for what is required to send a patient up to the ICU. I do not recall ever seeing her follow the list. There is also a checklist that the nurse follows before a patient goes into surgery. The problem here was that Sherry is faced with so many checklists, she needs a checklist to make sure she follows all the checklists! She is demonstrating her smarts by prioritizing. Given her deep understanding of the department and her patients, the time spent reading a checklist could sometimes be better spent in other ways.

Training Nurses

One major area that we try to prepare nurses for the demands of the profession can be found in nursing schools and the licensing of a new nurse. If fact, this is where much of the information overloading begins.

My journey as a nurse began on that first day of an EMT class. In hindsight, if there was an ideal way to train for nursing, this would be the route that I followed. As an EMT, you meet the patient in their homes or on the streets where they have had an accident or a medical crisis. You get to see patients "in their native habitat," such as their home or workplace, to get a fuller understanding of their lifestyle and who they are as people. I'm not saying the EMT experience was ideal because it was my path. Sometimes, with hindsight, you realize that the choices made in this case were the best. After my EMT program, the first ambulance company that got my resume, the one in my hometown, hired me. That is where I found myself at a patient's side within a couple hours into my first shift. This was about the lowest level of healthcare that made me the primary healthcare provider of that patient, a surprisingly high level of responsibility for someone with a mere 120 hours of training. Smarts also applies to EMTs, as I recognized a couple years later.

While in that job, I took the paramedic's anatomy and physiology class. This was not because I wanted to go that route, but people learn in iterations. We don't learn everything at once. We all need to get our information piece by piece. In this case, I got a little bit of the sciences until, a few months later, I was in my first pre-nursing class at the junior college. On the first day, trying to get admitted to the anatomy class, I put my backpack on the pile of plastic sheeting next to me. Another student looked at me strangely. "That's the cadaver," she told me. Oops. I took my backpack off of the dead person. And changed seats.

Nursing prerequisites can be summarized as lots of science with little context in which it is used. Medications taught in pharmacology are presented as names. The short, easy to remember ones are the trade names that manufacturers hope you will remember after their patent has expired. The long, complex, generic names are the ones the old patent holders hope you will not be able to remember so you order the trade names.

Nursing school was a life experience in itself. Other nurses advised me to sit in the back and keep my mouth shut, because some instructors do not like students with experience. That turned out to be true in my case. My case was typical in that every step of the way, some of my classmates went away. They did not pass a test or realized that nursing was not for them. Every step in the process involves filtering based essentially on book knowledge. While there has been much debate over

76

what a nurse currently practicing should know, there has not been much of a look back at those who never became a nurse to see if the supply chain is appropriate or fair. Imagine a person who wants to become a nurse but has not begun any of the college coursework. The filters to pass through include:

- Access to higher education
- Prerequisite classes, such as basic sciences
- Nursing school admission
- Nursing school
- Graduation exams
- National Council Licensure Examination (NCLEX)
- Licensing
- Background checks
- Hired into new grad position
- Preceptorship
- Retention

If one is coming from another country, there are also the additional hurdles of local labor laws, and government organizations to judge the equivalency of nursing education. The net result is that the discussion on nursing knowledge is focused almost entirely on those that have already passed through all of these filters and are licensed, employed, and practicing. Given the shortage of nurses and the evolution of nursing roles, we may want to look at the overall process and see if the end result is ideal for the nursing profession and for the healthcare system.

Every nurse in the North America goes through the rite of passage that is the National Council Licensure Examination (NCLEX). It is supposed to test the student on all that she needs to know to be a safe entry-level nurse. This test is created by the National Council of State Boards of Nursing (NCSBN), based in Chicago, representing all of the boards in the country. The NCLEX is required in all 50 states before a nurse can apply for a license to become an RN and has also been adopted by Canada.[11] Given the central role of the NCLEX in shaping the nursing profession, I was shocked to discover how little we know of whether it accurately reflects nursing knowledge and selects only those people that can work safely as new nurses.

Do an applicant's results on the NCLEX tell us anything about how well the applicant will be as a nurse? There is a vast amount of information built up around what kind of student does well on the test. That is easy to measure because we have large numbers of nursing students that are in exactly the kind of place that researchers can administer their questionnaires. Those variables are then compared with the NCLEX results. Unfortunately, it is not that simple. Nursing schools are judged based on their pass rates, which means they do not want anyone graduating from their program and failing the NCLEX. Better to not let them graduate. That has led to a pre-graduation exam that is modeled on the NCLEX. In other words, this is a test that measures how well you can take another test. Since most nursing programs require a passing score on an exit exam to graduate, I question the ethics of whether student nurses are being weeded out not based on the test that was meant to determine if they are safe but a test that is being used to promote a nursing school's reputation.

Again, does passing the NCLEX tell us whether the applicant is going to be a safe nurse? The NCLEX doesn't test for anything remotely similar to smarts. I don't see any way the NCLEX or any other written test taken in a quiet, safe room can equate to decision making in a busy, smelly hospital environment where lives are at stake. I couldn't find a single study that even attempted to match NCLEX scores with nursing performance. At the NCSBN conference, I posed this question to Doyoung Kim, the man responsible for developing the NCLEX, if there has been any such test of outcomes. He told me that such a research project is impossible because the data is the property of each state.[12] He was referring to was the fact that the NCLEX exam is the property of the NCSBN, but the results, including applicant demographic information and test scores, are owned by each state board. For example, in California the state board owns the data of applicants that took the exam in that state, even if the applicant came from elsewhere and plans to apply for a license in another state. I cannot put much stock in Kim's answer because, even if each state owns the data, there does not seem to be any major obstacle to getting permissions and access.

Scope of Practice

The picture I've painted so far is one of nurses overwhelmed in their workload and, in particular, their information load. I as a nurse cannot separate what I know with what I do. My actions will be judged, and only if there is a problem will I then be asked to justify my actions based on what I know. This leads to the final part of my discussion on smarts, which is where do we go from here? What can nurses do to control the information demands of the job and use smarts?

We cannot control how much information is out there. What we can control is how much information is held responsible for, and in what context. That means saying no sometimes. No to additional policies put out by our hospitals and the government regulators. In order to say no, a nurse needs the authority and control of her nursing practice, which, I have argued all along, is often lacking. Think of how many times in the past year you signed that you had completed some sort of "in-service training." Hospitals think that if they simply send a PDF to you by email and have you sign the training form, you should now know all that stuff—and they think they can hold you responsible for it. This is exactly what needs to stop. But there is more. It is not just about being defensive, but about taking control of our profession and using information to move nursing forward.

In the first week of nursing school, around that time that Erin was excited about learning lots of stuff that never did happen, I recall asking the instructor about our scope of practice. Specifically, we were being told nurses had a scope of practice that dictated what we could do, and to step out of that scope would lead to losing my nursing license. Doctors had their own scope, or so I was told. There was also mention of LPNs and nursing assistants, and others working in the hospital. I asked the instructor to lay out for us the scopes of all these key players so I could understand how the nurse fit in with these other clinicians.

The instructor looked at me with a slightly painful expression, and said, "that is a good question, and you need to know that information. If I just gave you the answer, you'll never learn for yourself. Go ahead and research that and let me know if you have any questions." I still remember her response. It meant she did not know the answer. Now, half jokingly, I use that as a piece of sarcasm. I asked my nephew, what is the diameter of the moon? He looked at me confused, so I explained. Any time someone asks you a question and you have no answer, just say, "that is an important question, and you need to know it. Look it up. If I just tell you the answer, you'll never learn for yourself."

Having been a nurse now for several years, I am amazed at how poorly we understand one of the key concepts of our profession, the scope of practice. We are judged by the minimalist standard of not making a mistake. One of the most serious mistakes a nurse can make is to go outside of our scope, but specifically into the scope of medicine. But what I want to address now moves beyond that, to what we nurses need to do to move our profession forward. Nurses are pushing the limits of our scope of practice, doing things that have historically been done by doctors. That leaves us in a dangerous situation, in which we can either retreat to that which is safely within our scope or try to grow as professionals.

In my July 2016 visit to the nursing board in one of the Rocky Mountain States, I witnessed a disciplinary hearing that was quite revealing. I've changed the name of the nurse and some of the details to protect anonymity, but the story is essentially the same.

That day, there was a disciplinary case involving Elena Forrest, a nurse practitioner. She was not present. A specialist in mental health, Elena had been charged with going beyond her scope at the urgent care clinic where she worked.

Confronted with a patient in pain, Elena gave the patient some ketorolac, a nonsteroidal anti-inflammatory drug (NSAID) similar to ibuprofen. The pain went away. But Elena was not authorized to prescribe (or, as some states call it, furnish) that particular medication.

The board members were debating the fate of her career. Some of them wanted Elena to lose her license. Some thought a probationary period of several months would be adequate. Others thought a simple warning would suffice. As I sat in the back of the meeting room and observed, it struck me that the reactions of others in Elena's case is a perfect example of how we nurses let our "scope" stop us from doing what is right based on our misguided perception that we need these limits.

Sure, nurses need to respect the law. And patient safeguards are important. But the fact is that ketorolac is a very safe drug, and Elena was familiar with it. How, I wondered, was patient safety an issue? But that's what boards do.

Elena's problems did not end there. To become an NP, she had applied to programs in Pennsylvania, and had to get an RN license in that state just to apply for the program. She ended up going to California for her NP schooling. Now that she was in trouble with her current state of practice, Pennsylvania took disciplinary action, so she needed to defend a license in a state where she had never lived and never worked. All of this started because the nursing scope of practice was holding back a good nurse from doing what was best for her patient.

Other nurses have a complex relationship with their scope, such as whether you work in an ED surrounded by doctors who can prescribe what is needed, or you are a nurse manager that is not medicating any patients but need to supervise those that do. Cynthia, as a hospital manager, has mixed incentive when it comes to her nurses adhering to their scope. She could let her nurses do more than what is in their scope, which may help patients get what they need even when there is not a doctor around. However, she will be judged by the hospital for any mistakes and allowing a nurse to go beyond her scope would be a severe infraction. Sherry is already working out of his scope on a regular basis, giving medications in the ED knowing that the doctors, whom she has known and worked with for years, will cover for her.

Where is our nursing scope of practice moving? Mostly toward the medical profession, taking on tasks that have historically been done by doctors. Part of this is because nurses have been working under the control of doctors, and thus this is the area that had the most familiarity. Another reason is money. That is where there is the best-compensated work. It would be odd if the nursing profession were actively seeking to take on tasks that would not get financially compensated. Although medicine is the area where the nursing scope has received the most attention, it is also moving into almost every other healthcare profession. There does not seem to be any other discipline where nursing has said no, we should not be pursing that. For example, nurses are now active in epidemiology, social work, mental health, and spiritual support. These are areas that already have established professions, such as social workers, psychologists, and chaplains. There's not nearly as much discussion when nurses assume tasks that would normally be done by, for example, social workers, as when nurses encroach on the practice of medicine.

For as important as the nursing scope of practice is, you would think there would be strong, concrete, and well agreed standards. Nothing could be further from the truth. In the United States, nursing is governed primarily at the state level. Already we can see that there is going to be at least 50 scopes and no promise of uniformity. Using California as an example, the board has a vague statement on what is nursing, equating that with the scope. It notes: "The practice of nursing means those functions, including basic healthcare, which help people cope with difficulties in daily living which are associated with their actual or potential health or illness problems, or the treatment thereof, which require a substantial amount of scientific knowledge or technical skill."[13]

It goes on to describe the independent functions, which is what we are most interested in. These are the things that a nurse can do without having to ask anyone. California's board states that the nursing laws "authorize direct and indirect patient care services that insure the safety, comfort, personal hygiene and protection of patients, and the performance of disease prevention and restorative measures."[14]

I found myself reading these passages, thinking there is wisdom and guidance to be found, if only I read it closely and think hard about it. Eventually, I realized that I am not missing anything. There is little to no useful guidance in state policies. Instead, what the law demonstrates is circular logic. Nurses do that which is which is within their scope, and the scope is that which nurses do. In the example of California, I see nurses can perform "disease prevention and restorative measures," and for all of the "actual or potential health or illness problems," the nurse can provide "treatment." That sounds like the nurse can do anything, and I know that is not true.

Guidance on how to determine what the scope is can either be sought in the state government's policies, or in how they are implemented and enforced. The government documents provide little information. Everyday practices offer much better guidance on what nurses actually do and how their scope has been interpreted.

Dan Tennenhouse, who teaches medical law at UCSF, gave me the clearest explanation that I have ever heard on what is in our scope. He advises that courts interpret the nursing scope as consisting of traditionally recognized nursing practices plus standardized procedures. In other words, instead of trying to collect a list of all the things that we are allowed to do, the courts look to see if nurses are performing that task, and then assume it is within the scope. Note how the process is the reverse of what logic would dictate. We look to the law for guidance on what we are allowed to do, and the law is just looking back at us saying, "if you nurses are routinely doing it, that must be part of your scope."

In my work in the ED, we had a patient who was constipated, and the doctor ordered a digital decompaction. In other words, someone needs to get their fingers in his rectum and scoop out the poo. The nurse refused, saying it was not in the nursing scope. Her logic was that nurses cannot do invasive procedures. This was interesting logic but utterly wrong. To begin with, she was just trying to avoid having to do the dirty deed. Second, if digital decompaction is invasive and thus outside our scope, how is it we do enemas? The doctor did not argue, because she was busy and fed up with this nurse. The doctor did it herself. Nurses often have strong incentives to either expand or contract our scope depending on the matter at hand. This nurse did not want to put her fingers up someone's rectum, so the scope contracted. Sherry needs to give medications and the doctor is busy elsewhere, so the scope expands. In all these cases, I realized that nurses simply haven't read the rules on our scope. That is not much of a concern because even if they did, it would not help guide them any.

Recognizing when and how the rules are going to get you in trouble can demonstrate nursing smarts. Refusing to do a digital decompaction even if it is in her scope was not going violate the rules, but it was an example of laziness. Giving a medication while expecting the doctor to cover her is a way some nurses demonstrate smarts by balancing the needs of the patient, the department staff, and her need to protect her license.

One of the most common ways of delineating nursing scope is to see where it goes into the scope of another profession: the practice of medicine. When a nurse is accused of doing something that is within the scope of medicine, she has little in the way of defense. This should not be the case. First, there is a large overlap in the scopes of nursing and medicine. Consider California's physician scope of practice: "The Medical Practice Act authorizes physicians to diagnose mental and physical conditions, to use drugs in or upon human beings, to sever or penetrate the tissues of human beings and to use other methods in the treatment of diseases, injuries, deformities or other physical or mental conditions."[15]

The concept of a scope of practice generally does not apply to medical doctors. They simply do not have any limits to their profession. If doctors have essentially no scope, and everything in the field of healthcare is potentially within their purview, then anything a nurse does is also the practice of medicine. So, the accusation that a nurse is "practicing medicine" is starting to look tenuous.

The nursing profession is growing and evolving, but our scope does not change much. These standards are inherently stifling because they only show what our current limits of practice are, not what they should be and not where they are heading. Some states have a process for interpreting disputes or answering questions from nurses about what is allowed. Some have well developed policies on interpreting changes, but boards usually do not have a legal process for expanding the scope. Nurses are warned never to go beyond the scope, suggesting a prudent nurse would stay well within the limits. That means the forces of regulation are pushing the profession backwards. If nursing is going to grow, the only way that can happen is, obviously, at the frontier. If nurses are advised by the boards not to go beyond their limits, progress is being discouraged.

The underlying assumption is that working within a defined scope keeps patients and nurses safe. That argument has not been properly tested in nursing, does not apply to doctors, and is inaccurate. Recall the earlier comments that one way to judge competency is that the nurse practices safely. Within the scope, the nurse still needs to demonstrate competence and could be found guilty of unsafe practice independent of the task being within her scope. This is the example of Elena. State nursing laws and the boards provide such little guidance that they create more confusion than direction. Actions that could improve patient safety are avoided out of fear of going beyond the scope. It is possible that something outside of the scope can be safely done by a nurse, but does not happen if a doctor is not available. No explanation is provided why the nurse needs to work under this limitation and not the doctor.

Oddly, we only hear about transgressions of nurses into medicine, as if that were the only boundary that matters. One almost never hears of nurses practicing psychology without a license, or dentistry, or chaplaincy. There's a lot of politics behind this phenomenon: some professions protect their turf, while others seem a lot more relaxed. Nurses have fought legal battles against doctors to get the right to perform many of the functions of, for example, a nurse practitioner. Not so with other professions. Look at the interest in spiritual services, yet there has not been the suggestion that a nurse is violating the scope of a chaplain. Mental health nurses seem to be doing a lot in common with mental health providers, but there does not seem to be the same reaction. In sum, professional turf battles and power dynamics explain what is going on with the nursing scope. Nursing smarts is how nurses adapt to the continuing challenges of the profession, taking on new roles where appropriate and safe.

Chapter 3 References

[*] Aiken *et al.*, "Education Levels …"

[2] Gawande, *The Checklist Manifesto*, 8.

[3] Schmidt and Rosenberg, *How Google Works*.

[4] Good, "Giving thanks …"

[5] Benner, *From Novice to Expert*, 25–26.

[6] Watson, " Clinical Competence."

[7] Abramson *et al.*, "Adverse Occurrences …"

[8] Kahneman, *Thinking, Fast and Slow*.

[9] Kahneman, Slovic, and Tversky, *Judgment Under Uncertainty*; Kahneman and Tversky, *Choices, Values, and Frames*.

[10] Bradley *et al.*, "Strategies …"

[11] NCSBN, "2013 Canadian RN Practice Analysis."

[12] Personal communication with the author.

[13] BRN, California, "An Explanation of the Scope of RN Practice."

[14] *Ibid.*

[15] *Ibid.*

4

From Errors to Just Culture

Sarah started her new job at the hospital ED after only six months in another ED where she was in a new graduate RN program. That opportunity was special, because few hospitals are willing to invest that much in new nurses. On her first day, the manager introduced her to her buddy nurse, an ex-paramedic, who was visibly annoyed at having to orient the new hire. "I'm going to do my job and you just ask if you have any questions," the "buddy" said as she quickly walked away. That was not unusual behavior for this particular department, which had a reputation for bullying. Still, Sarah was confident in her skills and willing to work hard.

As the first months rolled by, she realized there was a gap between her and the night shift's ruling clique of nurses. No manager was to be found on night shift, so these senior nurses ran the show. She wasn't one to spend social time with them, not that she was ever invited. As for the work, it was a constant struggle for all of them to keep up. ED nursing is quite simply a fast food business model, where you move as fast as possible and quality suffers. Then, a major error happened. A senior nurse brought unlabeled tubes of blood to the nursing station, the tubes got mixed with those of another patient, and the results came back showing the patient needed emergency dialysis. The doctor did not notice the difference between the patient in need of emergency dialysis and the other patient, and the wrong person got dialyzed. Wow, I cannot imagine a more serious mistake!

After that event, the nurses were all told to absolutely never take unlabeled tubes out of the patient's room. The tubes need to be labeled immediately after being drawn at the bedside. The senior nurse took this as they did most of what managers told them. Senior nurses ran their own show. A week later, the same thing happened. Unlabeled blood tubes were brought to the nursing station and mixed up with another patient. They caught the mistake this time. However, after that, the nurses were required to have a second nurse initial on the tubes for every blood draw. This was a major hassle, and it simply meant that after every blood draw, the nurse would walk around and ask the first nurse she found to initial off on the tubes. There was no double-checking going on, just a lot of initialing.

Around that time, Sarah made a mistake. The senior nurse that had mentored her as a new hire pointed to a newly arrived patient, moaning in pain, and told her to give the patient 4mg of morphine. Sarah, scrambling with her full load of patients and now taking on this additional one, grabbed 4mg of hydromorphine (Dilaudid). Moments later, the mistake was obvious. The patient was growing pale and breathing shallow. Because she was in the hallway, a passing doctor saw what was happening, and took action. The patient was given naloxone, and moved to the trauma room where she recovered from the medication error. Sarah was mortified by her mistake.

The managers were surprisingly understanding, and Sarah received verbal counseling and was required to be precepted for another month. Despite what the managers' intended, the night shift nurses had a different plan. After that, the buddy nurse that had previously been a constant source of support turned his back on her. No questions were answered and no advice would ever come from him. The group of senior nurses on night shift was now looking for every mistake Sarah made. It did not matter that other nurses were making mistakes. The only errors that would get reported from then on would be those made by Sarah.

Vancomycin was ordered for Sarah's middle-aged patient with an infection. The medication would need to be reconstituted, and she wanted to make absolutely sure there would be no mistakes, so she consulted another nurse who, although she had enough seniority to hold some sway in the department, was not among the power brokers. She reconstituted the vancomycin in 250ml of normal saline. Sarah proceeded to hang the medication. That is when one of the senior nurses went in to double check. It should have been 500ml of normal saline, not 250ml. There is a risk of a reaction when giving vancomycin, known as "red man syndrome," and that is why this antibiotic gets reconstituted in the extra large volume of normal saline. The senior nurse who caught the mistake immediately turned around, walked out of the room, and reported it to a manager. The senior nurse had not checked the patient, and neither did the manager. Neither of them told Sarah to stop running the vancomycin. The manager did not seem concerned that the other nurse had been the one to use wrong size saline bag, or that the nurse discovering the mistake did not check the patient or stop the infusion. From that point on, it would just be a matter of time before the next error would cost Sarah her job.

On the issue of medication errors, some mistakes are minor, and others may harm a patient's safety, but medication errors are treated more seriously than any other type of mistakes. Accusations of medication errors, and safety errors in general, are the weapons of choice for bullies, a point that is introduced in this chapter and elaborated upon in the next chapter.

Medication management is part of an overall safe nursing practice, and the patient's health is paramount. There are really two issues here: patient safety and a nurse's wellbeing, her ability to do her job free of intimidation from the hospital and her fellow clinicians. It is about allowing the nurse to focus on what is best for patient care and not what looks good in the documentation or in the hospital's performance reports. One approach to managing errors is known as *Just Culture*, based on the idea that nurses are humans and we all make mistakes, but in order to learn and improve, we cannot punish someone for making an innocent mistake.[1]

Medical errors have been in the popular press, scaring the public into thinking they are taking great risks when they go into a hospital. Martin Makary, a doctor at John Hopkins University, and research fellow Michael Daniel, declared medical error to be the third leading cause of death in the U.S.[2] This was a non-peer-reviewed article based on different accounting systems for large scale, epidemiological studies. Nurses are hardly the only targets for these accusations, but we are in the middle of this issue. When you look at the attention paid to medication errors compared to everything else that affects patient safety, there are major anomalies. The amount of potential harm done to patients does not result in consistent policies, and the brunt of these disparities falls onto nurses.

If the consequences of handing drugs were a positive attraction to becoming a nurse, it would be understandable that these special expectations would be part of the bargain. That is not the case. When asked why they became nurses, it is hard to imagine any nurse would respond that she enjoys handing controlled substances. There is simply not much fun in that, just responsibility. I have not seen any indication that anyone entered the healthcare field with the hope of having greater access to drugs. In other words, all of the challenges of handling drugs are things that nurses did not choose and only impede their ability to provide good patient care.

Medication Errors

Of all the standards and expectations made of nurses, perhaps none is so specific and, arguably, so unrealistic, as handling medication errors. Whereas the entire healthcare team has a duty to protect patient safety, and everyone involved in the provision of medications has a duty to ensure its accuracy, the nurse is inordinately judged and disciplined. Part of the issue is that patient safety is a major concern, and with medical progress comes increasingly fragile patients. The flip side to that is the frustration felt at the lack of further progress in patient outcomes. We saw dramatic improvements in life expectations and quality of life with the advent of sanitation and antibiotics. Since then, further advances have been much less dramatic, and the frustration has been landing to a significant degree on nurses. Lucian Leape, a doctor at Harvard, who is called the godfather of patient safety, noted about the amount of medical errors that affect patient safety and asks, "How much of a problem is patient safety? The unsettling fact is that no one knows."[3] Discussing the politics and financial aspects are often avoided, but the reality is that hospitals face multimillion-dollar settlements for any alleged errors—a large incentive for fixing the problem.

The modern patient safety movement has been traced to the 1991 Harvard Medical Practice Study in the *New England Journal of Medicine*, which found 3.75 percent of hospitalized patients suffered an adverse event (injury due to treatment, not disease), and that 14 percent of those injuries were fatal.[4] Another major report, the Institute of Medicine's (IOM) *To Err Is Human*, set the agenda for organizational and systemic changes as the preferred solution to medical errors, noting these are the most common single preventable causes of adverse events. The healthcare community is interested in all aspects of patient safety, but I treat the matter of nurses and medication errors as a case study to better understand the wider problem.

The typical first step in understanding medication errors is to look for the root cause. *To Err Is Human* states that instead of assigning blame on an individual, we need to look at organizational causes of errors and address those. That is disingenuous because systems are judged by how well individuals perform. If errors still occur, it is the fault of either an individual or the system. Either management should change the system, or the individual is at fault. Some nurses are making mistakes that are unacceptable, and some nurses are making mistakes that resulted from poor systems. Separating the two requires a wisdom that is truly a challenge. If the system is at fault, then one or more managers may be held accountable, but that rarely happens. For all the nurses that have been disciplined for medication errors, I am hard pressed to think of any supervisor or executive losing her license for a mistake.

Nursing management is mostly about assessing the quality, strengths, and weaknesses of employees. No system is capable of making every nurse competent and skillful. However, the idea that we need to look at the system provides little guidance on this matter. An incompetent nurse may have made an error that was the fault of the system, and a good nurse may have made an inexcusable error. Management discussions of errors and patient safety often refer to "never events"—something so bad it should never happen. In reality, good people can make amazingly bad decisions.

Consider the case of a parent leaving a child in the car on a hot day. Many assume that no parent could do that by accident, and it must have been done on purpose. However, Gene Weingarten won a Pulitzer Prize for his work showing how those people who have made this error and lost their child came from all walks of life.[5] This shows how everyone is at risk for making horrible mistakes, but nurses operate in an environment where they are particularly prone to this. Instead of looking for root causes of errors, we have a chicken-or-egg problem in which systems contribute to errors, but an individual error is always made by an individual. In other words, an error never just happens out of nowhere. Given all the double checks, documentation, and accountability in a hospital, there will always be someone there at the patient's side, catching the blame. Once you identify a person to blame, the situation becomes complex.

At the system level, the first thing that becomes apparent is that where you look for the problem is where you'll find it. Just looking at the sources of errors, there are lots of causes in all parts of the system.[6] Medication administration follows a cycle beginning with the doctor's assessment, diagnosis, and prescription of a medication. That prescription is processed by the pharmacy department and then returned to a nurse, who administers the medication. Most of the process is outside the control of the nurse, yet the research on this matter seems to emphasize the nurse's role.

Ignoring for the moment all the errors that occur outside the realm of the nurse's control, how do I know the prevalence of medication errors? Measuring errors has proven to be elusive despite a large, sophisticated research project. There are two commonly used definitions of *medication error*. One study defined it as "a deviation from the physician's medication order as written on the patient's chart."[7] Another definition is the American Society of Hospital Pharmacists' (ASHP) taxonomy of errors.[8]

- Prescribing
- Omission
- Wrong time
- Unauthorized drug
- Improper dose
- Wrong dosage-form
- Wrong drug-preparation
- Wrong administration-technique
- Deteriorated drug
- Monitoring

- Compliance
- Other

What we see here is that what is considered an error varies widely. For example, giving a medication that was prescribed, but the doctor made a clinical mistake, may be considered an error or not. There are errors of omission, in which a medication was missed, and errors of commission, in which a medication was given but in error. An "opportunity for error" included any dose given plus any dose ordered but omitted. Add up the medications ordered plus all the unordered doses given, and you get the "total opportunities for error." How far the study goes back to check if there were errors prior to the nurse's involvement also varies widely. When I was a new nurse, I once pulled out a medication because the system was not clear if this was a unit dose or a multiple unit bottle. When I pulled out the medication, a senior nurse told me it was the wrong medication, and the mere fact that I had pulled it up in our automated pharmacy system would qualify as a medication error.

Medication error detection is done by three main methods: chart review, incident reporting, or direct observation. Chart reviews involve looking at the documentation to see whether the doctor prescribed a medication correctly, whether the pharmacy delivered the drug correctly, and whether the nurse administered it correctly, as documented. The key part here is that we only know what was documented. It is quite possible that I did the right thing but documented it incorrectly or did the wrong thing and documented it as if I did it correctly. Direct observation studies involve the researcher walking around the clinical setting watching me do my job. Needless to say, the effect of direct observation on my behavior is inevitable. Incident reporting, the weakest of the three methods, looks at official reports of medication errors. These may be done by the nurse on a voluntary or involuntary basis, and they may be anonymous or not. Supervisors or the hospital also generate reports; these tend to be mandatory for any errors encountered by the mangers.

Nurses are smart people, and I am constantly amazed at how they can game the system to meet whatever management standards they are presented with. When management wanted all of the nurses to co-initial on the blood tubes, the nurses simply asked each other to sign off on each other's tubes. Electronic information systems allow us to change the time that a medication is given. Even if it is charted later, and I change the time of administration, there is almost no way they can confirm what actually happened. The more hospitals try to document every detail of me giving medication, the more errors there are going to be in the system. The only way around this is if I spent my shift catering to the needs of the documentation, and not the needs of the patient.

Given this situation in which medication errors are almost impossible to measure accurately, it should be no surprise that those who have tried to measure it do not agree on what is going on. One of the more thorough studies done found 20 percent of medication administrations had errors.[9] They included 36 hospitals and supervised nursing facilities in Atlanta and Denver areas, in which a nurse followed the medication nurse. The errors were reviewed by pharmacists for the potential harm to a patient, and of the errors, only 1.5 percent were deemed even possible adverse drug events. Not to make light of any medication error, but telling the public there is a .03 percent error rate (that's 1.5% of 20%) is not nearly as frightening as 20 percent.

But that's a very high rate of errors when the nurse knows she's being watched, and she knows exactly what they're looking for. Many hospitals declined to be part of the study, stating they were worried they would fare poorly. This was essentially an admission that those hospitals would have a worse score than what was eventually found.

Were the error rates found in this study an anomaly? Hardly. Results from numerous studies consistently show high error rates. Another study focused on nurses that administered IV medications, a high-risk event, and found they made errors half the time.[10] In a review of forty studies, chart reviews were found to have major errors in 0 to 88.5 percent of studies, and computer monitoring found major errors in 0 to 50.5 percent.[11]

Looking at the details of these studies, one can see lots of cases where the true error rates should be even higher, but not many in which they should be lower. For example, when British nursing scholar Jill Gladstone tried to measure errors an English hospital, she had to omit the registry nurses (referred to as bank nurses in the UK) for methodological reasons.[12] Those nurses new to a hospital are going to be unfamiliar with the process, and probably more likely to make errors. It would be hard to imagine a scenario in which the less experienced nurses would have lower error rates.

To appreciate fully just how much we are under-reporting errors, consider an online reporting form offered to NICU nurses to voluntarily and anonymously report medication errors.[13] Over the three years the system was in place, they received more than a thousand reports, of which serious patient harm was reported in 2 percent. This system was anonymous and voluntary, so there was little pressure to hold back on reporting. I'm going to assume that a nurse makes one error per shift— a conservative number for a high acuity department such as this. The number of errors reported was only 0.5 percent of all errors theoretically occurring. The differences in reported errors are massive, and they're the tip of the iceberg.

Controlling Medication Errors

So far, I see lots of errors and very little idea exactly how common they are. Only a tiny percentage of the errors are serious from a medical view, but that does not mean they are minor given the politics and the optics. Hospitals cannot appear to err on the side of not doing enough when it comes to preventing mistakes. What efforts are being made to control medication errors and how successful have they been? We have a very poor understanding of long-term trends in medication safety, and I could not find any study that followed nurses over a period of time to see how things changed. Programs to reduce errors have generally been less than a stunning success. Some attempts to reduce errors seem to show success, but many others made things worse.[14] The introduction of electronic health records led to a reduction of medication errors between 13 and 99 percent.[15]

A longitudinal study that identifies individuals would shed some light on whether bad nurses are the cause Imagine, though, the issues that would arise if nurses in a hospital department knew they were being watched for errors before and after some intervention such as training or procedures. The observation effect would make this study invalid from the outset. Even if the intervention were at the organizational level, they would still need to control for the personnel involved. Again, this would be a futile endeavor.

Another possible explanation for the large number is the nature of patient stays in hospitals. In Britain, a few decades ago the average patient stayed in the hospital for over two weeks.[16] Patients are now staying for much shorter periods of time and thus generating more turnovers. There are higher acuities combined with pressures to get patients discharged. In sum, the hospital environment seems to be more stressful and demanding.

Clearly, there are challenges in measuring the prevalence of errors. But how can we control mistakes? I see the problem of cause and effect. If nurses fear punishment, they will not report errors. Nurses are not willing to report on each other or on themselves. Half of nurses surveyed did not report medication errors for fear of punishment.[17] A Utah pediatric hospital's infant unit was surveyed, and 15 percent said they *never* saw any medication errors.[18] In another case, when nurses were asked what constitutes a medication error, and why a nurse might not report something as an error, they found the following reasons that nurses might deem an error does not qualify as a reportable:[19]

1. If it's not my fault, it's not an error.
2. If everybody knows, then it is not an error.
3. If you can put it right, then it is not an error.
4. If a patient has needs that are more urgent than the accurate administration of medication, then it is not an error.
5. If it is a clerical error, then it is not an error.
6. If an irregularity is carried out to prevent something worse, then it is not an error.
7. If none of the above applies, then the caregiver would call it an error.

Why are nurses not reporting errors? Most believed some errors were not reported due to fear of management's reactions.[20] These fears are probably well founded. In one of the best histories of medical errors, nursing scholar Kristine Karleson notes that the U.S. lawyers' association wanted mandatory reporting, but was opposed by the American Hospital Association and American Medical Association.[21] This leads to a question: What is hospitals' vested interest when it comes to reporting medication errors? You might assume that hospitals want thorough reporting of all errors, but I think that would be naïve. Consider the possibility that management has a vested interest in underreporting of medication errors. While a large percentage of nurses are not reporting errors, the studies I found did not mention any concerted effort of management to increase reporting. While almost everyone in the healthcare field is claiming that we should report errors, I don't see a lot of serious action to support this.

One of the most important changes to the way we as a society and in the nursing profession handle errors is known as *Just Culture*. It is a policy and a management philosophy based on the fact that humans are inherently error prone, and it is unjust and unwise to punish individuals for every mistake. *Just Culture* does not mean that errors are acceptable, but that there is a difference between honest mistakes that occur once, and those mistakes that are repeated or based on negligence.[22] I was attending the Washington State Board of Nursing's meeting on March 14, 2015, when Linda Burhans, of the North Carolina Board of Nursing, gave them a lesson on *Just Culture*. North Carolina's *Just Culture* policy provides guidance on what needs to be reported to the board, and what does not. This includes a "Complaint Evaluation Tool" in which a hospital can generate a score based on whether the mistake was human error, at-risk behavior, or reckless behavior.*

Hospitals struggle to decide if a mistake is reportable. If they fail to report something, it can reflect poorly on the hospital and allow an unsafe nurse to continue her practice. Report things that could be handled at a lower level, and that violates the nurse's right to just treatment, and intimidates others from reporting. When Burhans was speaking, the question was asked about how to change the culture and systems. Most states have a system in which all errors may be litigated, and failure to report can be a crime. Applying the *Just Culture* model may create liability for hospitals for failure to report. There was no good answer to that question.

I've seen many cases of nurses that reported medication errors or got caught making mistakes, and not being punished. These were sometimes handled according to the principles of *Just Culture*, and other times managers were simply too busy or uninterested to pursue the matter. Jasmine was a new nurse in a pediatric ED, and the doctor ordered prednisolone (a liquid) for an adolescent boy. She gave the patient prednisone tablets, thinking it was the same thing, but there are some distinct differences. The doctor was busy, as always, and when he saw this, called Jasmine aside and said, "You know, this is a med error." She just looked at him, waiting for whatever he may say next. And then he just walked off. That is was it. No error report was filed, and nothing

---

* See HCBON.com.

more was said of this. He could have reported it, and so could she. In this case, the doctor figured he made his point, and there was not much benefit to filling out report forms.

In another case, one of Cynthia's nurses Jake had given tamoxifen, a cancer drug, to a patient, with no complications. Jake had done everything correctly, and the patient tolerated the drug well, with one problem. As a cancer drug, the rules of this state require that the nurse be certified as an oncology specialist, which he was not. He simply did not know of this particular rule. Cynthia filed the reports, noting that the pharmacists had given him the tamoxifen without hesitation or warning of its special requirements, and the medication itself included no labels about it requiring special handling. She noted how this was a systems problem, and so Jake, instead of being punished, was congratulated for bringing this issue to the attention of management.

Part of the problem with medication error reporting comes from the fact that nurses are only one part of the supply chain from doctor to patient. If you look at them as part of this system, you may see the effects of organizational dynamics. Anne-Marie Brady, a nursing scholar, showed how numerous errors occur in medical reconciliation.[23] Medication reconciliation is when you check all of the medications patients are prescribed and ask them whether they *are* taking them—a process typically done when apatient arrives at the hospital or changes departments. Lots of errors are happening when this reconciliation is done. Yet imagine the RN, trying to decide how much faith to put into that medication record, and follow it diligently. If the record is known to be accurate, there is an incentive to follow it diligently. If you know the patient's medication orders are inaccurate, the incentive is then to do the opposite. Why follow to the letter something that you know has a lot of errors? The solution to this problem is not always clear. If you review the medications routinely, the chances of finding and correcting errors need to be greater than the chance of creating a new error. The realities of the clinical setting need to be considered. How many people that are perfectly lucid can give you a complete and accurate account of all their medicines, including dosages? Now imagine how many people far from lucid or knowledgeable are being asked what their medications are.

If the errors are all being made at administration, that puts the pressure on the nurse. But if the errors are being made earlier in the chain of events (prescription, processing, etc.), does that make things any easier for the nurse? Actually, no, it makes them harder. The nurse as the patient's advocate needs to look at the medication orders and constantly ask herself, does this make sense? If she knows there are errors in these orders, now she needs to second-guess the orders themselves rather than just focusing on administering the drugs.

The studies have mostly sought to identify as many errors as possible, yet common wisdom tells us that if you are looking for something hard enough, you are going to find it. If you want to find lots of medication errors, chances are, that is what you are going to find. Imagine if every nursing assessment was broken down into every piece of the process. One assessment at the beginning of the shift could easily hit a hundred data points. Imagine if those were being recorded and every assessment that turned out to be in the least bit inaccurate was deemed an error.

Medication errors have been declared to threaten patient safety, yet only about 1 percent of those errors are serious. What of the other 99 percent? The simple act of measuring something generates a cost and creates new errors. I did not see any consideration for the cost effectiveness of measurements. For example, one study gave nurses a scenario in which the patient missed a noon antibiotic dose because he was in x-ray for three hours.[24] To adhere to strict medication error control, one needs to take a nurse out of the unit, go to x-ray, and administer the medication. Taking that RN out of the unit is disruptive. Does that mean a nurse not familiar with the patient should give the medication? Or the nurse who is familiar with the patient does it, but now leaves her other patients with another nurse who is not familiar with them? The point is, reducing errors creates additional costs, and there has been little discussion of a cost/benefit analysis. No hospital could stand the publicity that would arise if it tries to save money by balancing the needs of patient safety with any perceived tolerance of medication errors.

Imagine a spectrum with two extremes on recording of medication administration. At one end, the hospital requires every single detail of medication administration, down to the expiration date of the syringe used, through documentation of patient's response to every single drug, and countersigned by a second nurse. In other words, a situation in which the nurse's time is being taken up doing nothing but giving medication according to exhaustive protocols. At other end is the near complete lack of any measurement. Nurses are given prescriptions that they are free to follow or not, and anything documented is appreciated but not required. Given the ethical bearing of the profession, what would nurses end up doing? These are purely hypothetical situations, but elements of both cases have been found in various clinical environments. The professional ethos of nursing does not require an order to give medications accurately and document appropriately. The nurse's own standards determine that. Yet on the other extreme, mandates to follow more and more explicit and detailed rules and standards are—not surprisingly—resulting in more errors.

Martin Johnson, a British nursing scholar, touches on this idea, but instead of a spectrum, he lays out two value systems: bureaucratic and professional. The table that follows, adapted from Johnson's article, provides an overview of his perspective.[25]

Bureaucratic nursing values	Professional nursing values
Procedure should be carried out in the way laid down	Procedures should be modified in response to patients' needs
Nurses should have little or no discretion in case they make mistakes	Nurses should be professionals responsible for their own practice
Nurses shouldn't make mistakes	One can improve only by acknowledging mistakes
Higher authority in the structure legitimizes actions	Rational argument legitimizes actions

This gives a hint at why nurses are being challenged with standards that have not resulted in the desired outcomes. None of the studies I looked at discussed what happens when nurses are found to have made errors, yet the evidence on underreporting make it clear that the response is not, as the IOM study states, to look for system's solutions. When a nurse is accused of making an error, the stress of the clinical environment is likely a major cause, to be discussed in a later chapter. Yet that excuse is not always met with much understanding.

Doctors, pharmacists, and managers do not seem to be getting disciplined for errors like RNs are. We do not have a good comparison on error rates between professions because the standards are so different. Doctors are also being held accountable for errors, and what affects them will also affect nurses. Lucian Leape, the "godfather of patient safety" mentioned earlier, notes that doctors work in a culture of "autonomous individual performance" that is contradicted by the complexity of the healthcare industry.[26] The doctors in the hospital environment work more in a team-based system, but play a distinctly different role. Any explanation for nurse medication errors must explain how we work in that context. Consider one example of how doctors and nurses are both making an error, yet hospitals accept this practice on a daily basis. Doctors sometimes "cover" nurses when prescribing medications. For those readers not in the healthcare field, this refers to the practice in which a nurse will give a medication, assuming the doctor will write the prescription after the fact. This may be done when the nurse feels certain the doctor will write that prescription, of if the nurse feels the doctor will acquiesce to the nurse's request that the prescription be written. However, doctors are not allowed to do this. There is nothing in the law that allows an RN to give a controlled substance without a valid prescription, and there is nothing that allows a doctor to cover an RN. In essence, the doctor is committing a crime whenever she covers the nurse.

As the anecdote about Sarah illustrates, bullying thrives in this environment in which errors are constantly happening. An easy way to bully a nurse is to report any errors, which is going to happen if one simply waits long enough. Documented errors cannot be ignored by management, which is then forced to take some sort of corrective action. If multiple errors are reported, the bully can then easily have the nurse disciplined, all without the usual signs of harassment. The entire process is entirely legal, and the victim has no defense. Even if the relationship does not appear to be antagonistic, the mere existence of what Cosby and Croskerry, both emergency medicine doctors, refer to as a *power gradient* has been shown to create the risk for errors.[27] Those with less authority do not always speak up to prevent errors, or when they do, their concerns are not addressed. The scenario they cited was between doctors, in which the underling was correct and the superior (a senior doctor) was wrong. Power gradients work within professions and between professions. We work in an environment of uncertainty, where every clinician can make mistakes and be challenged. There is a complex dance of uncertainty, power, and the potential for error playing out while the clinician is trying to protect the patient but also protect her job.

Chapter 4 References

[*] Marx, "Patient Safety and the 'Just Culture'."

[2] Makary and Daniel, "Medical Error."

[3] Leape, "Scope of Problem and History of Patient Safety."

[4] Brennan *et al.*, "Incidence of Adverse Events and Negligence ..."

[5] Weingarten, "Fatal Distraction."

[6] Keers *et al.*, "Causes of Medical Administration Errors in Hospitals." The article identified 54 studies published between 1985 and May 2013.

[7] Allan and Barker, "Fundamentals of Medication Research Error."

[8] AHSP, "ASHP Guidelines on Preventing Medication errors in Hospitals."

[9] Barker *et al.*, "Medication Errors Observed ..."

[10] Taxis and Barber, "Causes of Intravenous Medication Errors."

[11] Manias, "Detection of Medication-related Problems in Hospital Practice."

[12] Gladstone, "Drug Administration Errors."

[13] Suresh *et al.*, "Voluntary Anonymous Reporting of Medical Errors ..." This study surveyed 739 nurses in the Vermont Oxford Network, with reports received 2000-2003.

[14] Keers *et al.*, "Impact of Interventions ..."

[15] Ammenwerth *et al.*, "The Effect of Electronic Prescribing ..."

[16] Audit Commission, "A Spoonful of Sugar."

[17] Brady *et al.*, "A Literature Review ..."

[18] Antonow *et al.*, "Medication Error Reporting."

[19] Baker, "Rules Outside the Rules for Administration of Medication."

[20] Gladstone, "Drug Administration Errors."

[21] Karleson *et al.*, "Medical Error Reporting in America."

[22] Marx, "Patient Safety and the 'Just Culture'."

[23] Brady, Anne-Marie *et al.*, "A Literature Review ..."

[24] Gladstone, "Drug Administration Errors."

[25] Johnson, "Drugs and Discipline." The author refers to these as British bureaucratic nursing values and British professional nursing values, but I see no difference in how they view it and how we in the United States view this issue.

[27] Leape and Berwick, "Five Years After ..."

[28] Cosby and Croskerry, "Profiles in Patient Safety."

5

From Bullying to Solidarity

Gina, an ICU nurse, moved from the Arizona countryside to the West Coast to begin a new life with her son. She soon got a job with one of Central City's major hospitals, noted for its innovative surgical techniques. The manager at the time was holding the position on an interim basis, and the two got along well. Gina enjoyed the challenging new position and living in a city.

The first year in the job went well, but then management changed. The interim manager was replaced by someone who needed to make a mark for herself and was under pressure from the hospital to make changes. Gina looked around at the staffing to make sense of what was happening. The certified nursing assistants (CNAs) had a union and were well organized. The RNs did not have a union, which was a little odd considering most other nurses in this region were unionized. Gina made a point of working well with everyone on the team, whether that meant the doctors, CNAs, or other RNs, but she also was ultimately held responsible for the patient care. That put her in an awkward position with the CNAs: She was not their supervisor yet accountable for the work they performed.

One CNA who worked with Gina on a regular basis was not always attentive to her patients, and Gina did what she could to make up for the shortcomings. One day, she called the CNA aside and pointed out that the preparations for surgery that needed to have been done were not. If the CNA could not do it, Gina would, if she had had the time and notice. Instead, the CNA did not do what was expected, and now it fell on Gina to rush things along. The CNA simply responded, "You're not my boss!"

This is where the union membership comes in. The CNA was a union member, and the managers clearly feared them. Call it respect or call it fear, but there was a lot of power behind the CNAs. They would not tolerate what they perceived as abuse. In this case, Gina was called into the manager's office and told her interpersonal communications style was abrasive. Worse, the CNA was an ethnic minority, and Gina was white, so there was a racial issue. This hospital had recently lost a case in which a large group of people of color claimed discrimination and won in court.

At this same time, there was a fellow RN of Gina's who seemed to be getting groomed as the next manger. In one of the department meetings, he expressed enthusiasm for the coming changes, saying he had a lot of good ideas for "our" department. That is when the manager responded, "this is not 'our' department. This is my department. I am responsible for what happens here."

In the ensuing months, three RNs were fired from that department, all of them being senior nurses who had been earning more money. Gina was the next in line in terms of experience and thus earnings. She was told that she had not charted on pain, when in fact she had. Not in real time. The manager wanted charting done in real time. In the clinical environment, patient care should come first, then documentation. Hospitals are increasingly calling for real time documentation to deter gaming of the system and what they might call dishonesty. None of the other RNs in this ICU where being told to chart in real time, just Gina.

The next error was a missed stool softener. A patient did not get a stool softener on time. OK, that is, technically, a medication error. In the hierarchy of medication errors that can affect a patient's short-term health, this is probably close to the bottom. As if these clinical issues were not enough, she was also called into the manager's office to explain why she was friends with a particular doctors. Was this a friendship or was there something more going on? Gina was thinking to herself, "I'm an adult. He's an adult. Why is my employer even asking what we might be doing on our own time?" The manager said that the relationship, whatever it might be, was unacceptable. As it turns out, this doctor first noticed Gina because she was the only RN documenting an end of shift synopsis of the patient. The hospital told them to keep it short and factual. Gina was writing a paragraph or two painting a picture of what was going on. The doctor appreciated that, and that is why they were in contact with each other.

Seeing the writing on the wall, she left that job, as much as she had loved the hospital and clinical role, because an RN cannot afford to be fired from a job or get reported to the nursing board. She applied to the other hospital in the same city, part of the same network. She was told she would not be getting an interview. She was blacklisted. As she moved on in her career, she wondered what had gone wrong.

Often when I feel wronged, it's hard to face the fact that it's my mistake and not "theirs"—but not always. As I reflect on my experiences in other hospitals, and the stories I keep hearing from other RNs across the country, there is a trend. Some errors are legitimate, and some nurses are not safe, but there is also a lot of accusations of errors that are simply not true. They are not honest accusations but a symptom of something more problematic.

Gina contacted a lawyer and was surprised to hear that she is not alone. Many of the issues could not be litigated, like charting in real time or a late stool softener. But there were things that could be pursued. The lawyer being inundated with nurses from this hospital chain reporting that their time cards were being altered and they were being denied break time. Gina would show up half an hour early to check her patient's lab values and get a proper report. She would also stay afterwards to complete the documentation, long after she had clocked out. During breaks, she was not allowed to leave the floor because they would often come to her with questions and requests. Documentation time stamped after one has clocked out is hard to refute. Ironically, the things that mattered least to Gina's patient care were the things that could be litigated. And it was. And she won. The money gained was a pittance, but she made her point.

Nursing Reaction to Stress

Gina's story is an example of what many nurses are going through, even if the storyline plays out differently. The underlying cause of this is working in a highly stressful job for which there is a high demand but limited supply. This compels nurses to behave in ways that are counterproductive to their shared interests. Normally, a group of professionals that are in short supply would use that source of power top improve their working conditions. For example, at containerized ocean ports, a person can get killed working around those large metal boxes, so dock workers have pushed successfully for safety measures. That solidarity is not so common in the nursing profession. I am seeing this problem that must be overcome if nurses are to take control as a group of professionals, and not as individuals managing our own transactional relationships with employers.

Stress is found in all aspects of nursing, and in almost every part of life, to greater or lesser degrees. The acute care clinical environment is notorious for high levels of stress. This is important for a variety of reasons, some obvious, and some not so obvious. Stress is what helps some of us keep focused and motivated, but under the same circumstances, that same stress can incapacitate others. A person can only absorb so much stimuli, known as cognitive load.[1] Stress is the symptom that we are getting very close to—or have already reached—this limit, and any demands on us that go beyond this limit may not be manageable.

There are two types of stress: acute and chronic.[2] Acute stress is what happens in a very short span of time, usually related to an event or some change in circumstances. The feeling can go as quickly as it comes. Chronic stress suggests a feeling that is ongoing, which may not appear like a problem but the cumulative effects prove to be damaging. Nurses are faced with both. In Gina's case, there was the acute stress created by the patient care. The management keeping her under the microscope created chronic stress. Gina could not relax at any time, even after work. Long after she left the job, she was still suffering from the chronic effects of that stress.

There is a difference between the kinds of stress nurses face and that of other professions. A nurse must perform complicated, lifesaving skills and sophisticated intellectual processes, all while working under stress. Other professions are not being forced to make such decisions while under those conditions. For example, a pharmacist, while overworked, is not treating the patient, and only has the abstract notion of what the medications are being used for. Assisting hospital staff may be at the patient's side and also under some of the same stresses as the nurse, but they are not making the kind of life and death decisions that the nurse is.

Some nurses under stress seek support from others, and some distance themselves from the stress in order to get the job done. My preceptor told me that I could get help if needed, but warned, "You don't want to go to the well too often." In other words, nurses need to get their job done, and functioning in a stressful environment is part of that. I see this as an area where solidarity can have a positive difference in helping nurses work together and work more productively.

Here is a common phenomenon: The busier the nurse is, the more outlandish measures some patients take to get her attention. The things patients do to get attention prevent the nurse from making decisions based on what is appropriate for all of her patients, and it can also lead to bad clinical decisions. In one extreme case, a patient decided that the threat of a gun would help him get attention for his psychiatric issues.[3] As I read this in my local paper, the journalists—rather than showing the harm done to all hospital staff and the other patients—made that person brandishing a gun into something of a hero.

Isabel Menzies, a British nursing scholar, performed a classic early study on the role of stress in a hospital.[4] She worked at a facility that had a training program for nurses. These students were supposed to get six months of training before starting practicum, which would include study and work. As the demand for their labor began to overwhelm them, fewer and fewer nurses were able to complete their six months of training before they were simply put to work. Some managers in the hospital had the foresight to see the error of this and commissioned a study. What they found was so shocking that it changed the entire project. As they interviewed the nurses, both student and experienced, as well as management, they found a strong sense of being overwhelmed. This led to the famous article of Menzies in which she laid out defensive mechanisms nurses use to manage the situation.

The important point from the Menzies study was that when hospitals demand too much of their staff, consciously or otherwise, workers react as individuals and even as groups to manage the excessive demands. Often, this results in hospital goals not being met, frustration among the staff, and bad outcomes. Organizations have a few options in how to manage or control the stress, but they need to think through how individual workers react under these conditions. Healthcare is an inherently stressful profession, and the fact that the stress is concentrated in certain departments is impossible to avoid. There is no magical solution to take the stress out of nursing. If that were possible, most acute care nurses would leave the field. This is why we chose this line of work. The excitement and challenge that attract us is exactly that which drives others away. Therefore, we approach this issue more as a matter of balance, reducing the destructive aspects of stress such as bullying, while embracing the positive effects, such as high patient acuity, as a chance for nurses to make a difference.

The amount of stress nurses face should concern not only nurses and hospitals, but the general public, as well. A nurse's workload affects her ability to give safe patient care. Each additional patient per nurse increases the odds of mortality by 7 percent—that is, mortality within 30 days of admission.[5] Each additional patient caused a 23 percent increased risk of burnout for the nurse. This led to legal changes in California, where the state passed the first law to establish nurse-to-patient ratios. Ratios differ for various areas, but in the intensive care area, the ratio was set at 1:2, meaning, no intensive care nurse could have more than two patients. Soon after the nurse-to-patient ratio regulations went into effect, California's nursing Board reported being inundated with RN applicants from other states. Applications for nursing licenses increased, and vacancies for RNs at California hospitals plummeted.[6] Gina had worked in Arizona where, as a newly graduated nurse, she was given responsibility for 8 med-surg patients. In California, if she were working in the med-surg department, she would only be given a maximum of 5 patients.

Besides workload, nurses are faced with another well-recognized source of stress, known as *moral distress*. This arises when you know the right thing to do, but institutional constraints make it nearly impossible to pursue the right course of action.[7] Moral distress begins with an initial feeling of distress, such as when you see patient care not going as you believe it should. Then you feel reactive distress from not being able to do anything about it. The TV show *Nurse Jackie* was based on the theme of a nurse's struggle with substance abuse, who would break the rules when it was in the patients' best interest. Viewers seemed to feel a connection with this nurse whose moral compass could cut through the hospital bureaucracy.

When I was working in the pediatric ED, a nurse was struggling with the guilt of how she handled a doctor that wanted to discharge a young child that was still wheezing. This child's oxygen saturation was good, but his lungs sounded awful. The nurse wanted to see him admitted, but the doctor did not think that was necessary. For the rest of the shift, I could see this pained look on the nurse's face as she thought about how hard she should have pushed her case. In hindsight, I see how a lack of solidarity among the nurses led to this powerlessness vis-à-vis the doctor.

But the concept of moral distress can get tricky, since it assumes the person experiencing it was absolutely right that something wrong was going on. This is not always the case, however. I have seen countless cases in which nurses disagreed with each other or the doctor, and they felt their views were not just an informed opinion but a moral obligation. To back down would mean an injustice to the patient. You can see vehement disagreements among nurses and doctors over the care for the same patient, and everyone can't be right.

Along with stress comes the possibility of burnout, in which a nurse has pushed herself to the limit. Linda Aiken, a California nursing scholar, found lower rates of burnout in California compared to other states.[8] This lower rate likely reflects the benefit of staffing ratios, but even there, almost a third of nurses reported being burned out. However, the picture is mixed. Another study found new nurses among the most satisfied.[9] ICU nurses reported high levels of post-traumatic stress disorder (PTSD) symptoms,[10] but there were low levels of stress among another group of British ICU nurses.[11]

Gina's hospital chain wasn't trying to create stress *per se*. As she recounted her story to me, nothing suggested any personal animosity. They were trying to cut costs. Cynthia, the hospital manager introduced in an earlier chapter, shudders at the thought of her staff getting mistreated or discriminated against, yet she is also responsible for keeping costs down, enforcing the rules, and disciplining nurses when necessary. Even when a nurse has the best of intentions, we are working in organizations where individual choices are not resulting in collectively good outcomes.

Cynthia has been a manager for many years now and seems to have found a long-term strategy to cope with the job stresses that she faces. However, many other nurses have not been so fortunate. That is why we need to look at the bigger picture of how stress is playing out in the nursing profession, how nurses react to it, and how we need to resolve this. My first step is to look at some specific ways that nurses are reacting to the stress.

My concern for nurses like Todd, Gina, and Sarah, is that while they may be coping with the job demands for now, is it sustainable? Cynthia has been a manager for many years now and seems to have found a long-term strategy to cope with the job stresses that she faces. However, many other nurses have not been so fortunate. That is why we need to look at the bigger picture of how stress is playing out in the nursing profession, how nurses react to it, and how we need to resolve this. My first step is to look at some specific ways that nurses are reacting to the stress.

Bullying as Risk Management

Many nurses use stress as a tool of manipulation and use bullying purposefully to protect their positions and achieve their goals. Bullying is far from being an unconscious act from harried or overwhelmed nurses. When nurses lack solidarity in a department or an entire hospital, they often fill the power vacuum by bullying.

There seems to be something special about nursing that makes bullying more significant than in many other professions. The problem is not just in the U.S. but in many other countries, where it has also been referred to as mobbing, harassment, or lateral violence.[12] The topic is of particular interest because it involves some fundamental dynamics of how nurses interact and the social environment of the entire facility. It affects a nurse's ability to provide safe care, a manager's ability to understand what is truly going on in a department, and even a person's ability to hold her job. Communication, the life-blood of healthcare, is devastated because honest messages are lost amongst the lies, the scheming, and the silence. Nurses were asked what they wanted in a job, and what tradeoffs they would take. On average, they said they would forgo about 17 percent of their income for a work environment free from bullying.[13] That huge sum gives you an indication of how severe and widespread this problem is.

Bullying can lead to nurses becoming silenced.[14] That was Sarah's experience in her ED. She was the new nurse and tried to get along by not complaining. It didn't work. "When [bullying] occurs, all meaningful communication is essentially stopped."[15]

Bullying is not just a nursing thing. CNAs, such as the one who confronted Gina, are also being bullied. You might think that doctors, for all their power and authority, would be above bullying, but they are not. Bullying happens in other industries, and not just among healthcare workers.[16] But there has been surprisingly little research on bullying, especially in the nursing field.[17] In the few studies I found, the prevalence of bullying ranges widely, from 17 to 76 percent of nurses reporting that they had been bullied. Part of the reason for the wide range may be explained by the fact that there are inconsistent definitions and methodologies.[18] There is a question of whether women bully more or less than men, and whether there is a difference in the types of behaviors they use. Sandra Thomas, a nurse scholar writing on nurse anger, found that both genders are being victimized.[19] Janet Bickel is a nursing scholar and author of *"Why Do Women Hamper Other Women?"* She noted: "The turmoil resulting from feeling undermined or cut by a trusted woman seems to have more negative impact than women's conflicts with men."[20]

In studies on bullying among nurses, we only see what is going on among those who chose to stay or were able to stay in their jobs. Sadly, the vast majority of nurses like Gina, faced with the prospect of being fired or disciplined based on false accusations, switched jobs.* That means that the bullies were successful in their efforts. If a large percentage of bullied nurses are moving, and those who remain are still reporting bullying, then the prevalence of bullying is far greater than what we have measured.

To understand why it occurs, it is first necessary to figure out where it happens. Bullying "tends to be more common in settings where technical expertise is valued over interpersonal competence," according to nursing researcher Judith Vessey.[21] Bullying is also happening in nursing schools, so the dynamics I am describing seem to start early in a nurse's career. There is anecdotal evidence that bullying is more of a problem intra-professionally than inter-professionally,[22] as indicated by the incidence of bullying done by other nurses as opposed to non-nurses. The statistics just shown support the idea that most bullying is nurse on nurse.

The causes of bullying have been explained in a few ways.[23] There are attempts at biological explanations, which include things like hormones or genetic predisposition. There didn't seem to be much to be gained from this approach, since aggression at the biological level does

---

* This statistic seems to be the only one from a large-N study—that is, one looking for patterns in a large number of cases—in the United States in which the specific stated reason for leaving the job was bullying.

110

not explain how individuals work in an organization. Developmental models are similar to biological ones: they seem far removed from the problem. The two areas that have been applied with more focus are inter-personal and intra-personal. Among the major intra-personal explanations are drugs and alcohol, family dynamics, and personality issues. One of the most noted from this group is Jack's work on the silencing effect. Inter-personal explanations have been the most widely used, particularly the oppressed group theory (OGT).

Nursing scholar Susan Jo Roberts wrote a seminal paper on oppressed groups, claiming nurses also qualify as such.[24] Her ideological heritage came from Paolo Freire, a Brazilian educator who wanted to reform how children are educated, believing that a feeling of helplessness is what prevents the lower socioeconomic classes from gaining an education.[25] Roberts and others adapted this idea to explain bullying behavior among nurses as a reaction to being oppressed. The psychology of passive-aggressive behavior in nurses is due to their secondary/assistive role to doctors and relative lack of power, leading to nurses lashing out at each other.[26]

There are a few problems with the argument, both in its logic and the evidence for it. To begin with, Freire's work was based on a class of people, and specifically Brazil's poor. A profession is not the same thing as a socioeconomic class. For a Brazilian peasant to get out of her class is essentially impossible. Rare individuals do, but they are the exception. For nurses to qualify as an oppressed class, it means that they are stuck in that profession and cannot move. There is something forcing them to continue being nurses. Roberts's argument was not that nurses are part of a wider group of oppressed workers that span all the poor of America, but that we as a profession constitute that group. That means we are stuck as nurses and have as little chance of getting out of nursing as that poor person in Brazil has of getting out of poverty. The argument of nurses as an oppressed group is already looking weak, but it gets even weaker.

According to Roberts, doctors are the ones oppressing nurses, yet these doctors have a professional ethos of caring that is essentially the same as nurses. Does the nurse report to the doctor as her supervisor? No, nurses almost always report up a nursing chain of command, and doctors report up their own chain of doctors. If that nurse is reporting to her supervisor, who is also a nurse, and the doctor is oppressing them, where is the influence that would empower that? The doctors do not hire nurses and they do not fire nurses. The doctors do not write the performance evaluations of nurses. All of that's done by nurses. An organizational explanation of nursing behavior that has doctors oppressing nurses needs far more justification.

It has been well established that nurses have been under heavy control from doctors. That legacy continues. I've seen in some hospitals that doctors who do not like a particular nurse can get her fired even when the nursing management disagrees. On the other hand, I have seen the nursing management stand up to the doctors and exhibit nursing professionalism. Even if nurses face some degree of control by doctors, it doesn't come close to explaining how we translate that into bullying.

If the position of authority leads one to be an oppressor, what of all those people working under nurses? There are many, including LVNs and medical assistants. If nurses are acting out as a result of being oppressed, but the target is someone under them in the power structure, then it is the nurse who is now the oppressor. I thought it possible that Gina's relationship with the CNA was not as she described, but in fact that CNA felt like she was the one being oppressed. Why then is the oppressed group argument so persuasive? It puts the blame on someone else other than nurses. The doctors are the oppressors, and nurses are the innocent victims.

Interventions to reduce bullying have generally been unsuccessful.[27] To get solid improvement in this area, we need change that is not just transactional, such as having a no-tolerance policy and a list of sanctions, but change in the overall culture.[28] Attention has been shifted to nursing schools, hoping to cut off a vicious cycle by training nurses to deal with the bullying that is to come in their careers. Instead of trying to change the culture of incivility, hospitals are simply preparing their new nurses to survive in a hostile environment.[29] It is as if hospitals have given up on any attempts to stop bullying.

To get at the problem of bullying, it is important to consider the idea that bullying is a conscious decision to gain specific advantages. There is a reason the perpetrator is doing it, and there have been a lot of benefits gained in doing so. To reiterate the main theme of the book, nurses are overloaded and judged on unrealistic and contradictory standards. Mistakes are happening routinely, but rarely punished. It makes sense to protect yourself, and the best way is to make sure you are working with people who are your friends and can be trusted. If someone shows up in the department who cannot be trusted, the easiest way to get rid of her is to enforce the standards that nobody else adheres to. Think of bullying as risk management. If nurses do not use it against those they cannot trust, they could become the target themselves.

Common bullying tactics include accusing the victim of errors, typically affecting patient safety. If you accuse someone of a safety error, the hospital is required to investigate. Such an accusation cannot be simply dismissed as nurses squabbling among themselves. Once a nurse has been accused of one mistake, she is under the microscope, and other mistakes are guaranteed to be found. It does not take much to get her removed, all without a hint that the patient safety report was done as a bullying tactic.

Recall Bana, the registry nurse working with Sherry. Whereas Sherry was part of the nursing power structure, Bana could be sent away without hardly any justification. Her registry company wants to remain on good terms with the hospital, so when there is any conflict with the nurse, that nurse is simply reassigned, no questions asked. Nurses know this, so they are free to make an accusation knowing that it won't be questioned. Sherry would not do that, given per professional bearing, but it only takes one nurse in the department to get Bana removed.

Even if the management knew what was happening, the hospital would still need to investigate the safety issue, and the fact that a nurse reported it with ill intentions could not be proven. When you look at a mistake and try to determine if it is out of line with what other nurses are doing, that would mean investigating all the other cases in which no complaint was made. Clearly, that does not happen. When a nurse is accused of something, her actions are mostly compared with others who were also being investigated and, more often than not, from those found guilty of wrongdoing. Think of all the times a nurse was accused of something, and notice that her alleged misdeed is common practice among nurses.

Theresa Brown is a nurse with a PhD in English who wrote a fictional account of a typical nursing day. She notes in *The Shift* how she would decide whether to chart vital signs at the time they were taken, or when they were supposed to be done.[30] Here is a nurse that is apparently quite a good and conscientious one describing something—the falsification of documentation—that could get a person fired. She goes on to describe how the phlebotomist draws an extra tube but holds onto it for half an hour, as if it were drawn separately. Again, this is a behavior that is common practice, yet is a fireable offense.

I showed in the discussion on medication errors that nurses inevitably make mistakes, and they occur on a near constant basis in the acute care environment. In that situation, every nurse is at risk of being accused of something. Hospitals almost always fire a nurse rather than report her to the Board. Even if a nurse's mistake was roughly on par with the mistakes made by her co-workers, that may not help her once she is before the Board's disciplinary process. Even if she is exonerated, simply being sent before the Board or placed under probation will condemn her career.

If you want to get someone you do not like out of the department, the statistics show that most of the time the victim does not complain, and usually leaves. We often hear nurses say how much they would love to work in an environment free from bullying. But that is exactly why it works. If a department that is well paid and the workload is not too bad, we can expect bullying by a clique of nurses to protect that situation. They can choose who will be their future co-workers and eliminate others by strategic use of bullying. Solidarity is when nurses work together as professionals, but I see cliques as small groups of nurses protecting their personal interests against other nurses, harming the profession.

I worked a few shifts at Doctor's Medical Center in San Pablo, California, and there was no bullying going on. Great! No, it wasn't great. It was the most disorganized and dangerous place I have ever worked. Paper documentation on a patient would be left on the counter for me to pick up. That was their "filing system." Often there would be patients in one of my four beds, dumped there with no report. And I would find a patient gone, having been admitted upstairs or discharged, all without my knowledge. After four shifts, I called the manager to resign. No response from my call. I left four messages on the answering service of four different managers, no response. So I never went back. Two weeks later, I got a call from the accounting department, asking if I would please remember to sign my time sheets in the future. A couple years after this, the hospital shut down. Ironically, there was no bullying. We all got along rather well. Why? Because this job was so lousy, there was no incentive to bully.

Nurse managers are supposed to be the ones controlling the bullying, but they are also bullying and being bullied themselves. Hospital supervisors are usually busy and working under stress, so the time and effort needed to investigate and control bullies is only going to become a priority if it affects the department's operations. Given the current situation in which victims move instead of complaining, the prevalence of bullying is unlikely to change. I need to emphasize at this point that solidarity is about the profession, and that means nurses in management and non-management working together.

Bullying is not done in bursts of passion. It usually happens in a very cool, calculated, and premeditated manner. Even if nurses work in stressful conditions, look at all the examples of bullying behaviors: isolation, exclusion, gossip, denied opportunities. These are not things done in the heat of desperation by a nurse struggling to keep up with her workload. If anything, it takes additional time and effort to do some of these things. Gina's manager was auditing her charts, looking for any fault. Sarah's accusers, the senior nurses, were not lashing out in frustration. They had found a way to keep control of their department, and that was by selecting what nurses got to stay, and Sarah was not one they trusted.

The overall effect on patient care is clear. Any reports of medication errors, for example, beg explanation. If less than 1 percent of all errors end up getting reported, there needs to be an explanation for why that error was chosen and not any of the other 99. This has led us to a situation in which medication error reporting is essentially useless in determining the true rate, but it tells us a lot about power dynamics within a department. It becomes clear who runs the show and who does not.

When hospitals seek to end bullying behaviors such as insults or overt harassment, they simply cause the power leaders to shift tactics. Instead of open hostility, reports of patient safety violations will work more effectively, and with less effort on the part of the instigator. It has a double advantage in that the supervisors will be so distracted investigating the reported violation, they will have that much less time to address the root cause.

One other explanation of bullying has been learned behavior, in which nurses that were bullied later become the bully.[31] I do not see how that explains much. First, bullying is so common, almost every nurse is subjected to it. Since you have such a large pool of ex-victims, we are going to see a significant number of them become bullies. Second, it is suggested that bullying is passed on in the same manner as an abused child grows up to be the abuser. Much of the causal effect in nurse bullying is different. It is simply that a nurse sees how it can be useful for career survival, so some are going to use it, whether she was previous victims of bullying or not.

Hospitals as a Challenge to Nurses

Nurses mostly work in hospitals. There is a trend toward non-hospital employment, like clinics, nursing homes, or home care nursing, but these places employ less than half the nation's nurses. The years spent working in a hospital are the formative ones for a typical nursing career. This is where we get most of our acute care experience and work with a broad range of healthcare professionals to learn the big picture of how this system works.

Hospitals are inherently organized. They are institutions. Some are nonprofits; others are for-profit corporations. They are not just a group of people working together in a building. This is the fundamental difference between nurses and our employers. Hospitals do not need an excuse for presenting a unified front against outsiders. Leaders are paid to look after the organization's interests. In fact, everyone is required, as a term of employment, to look after the organization's interests.

Contrast this with the nurses. We are individuals that mostly work as individuals in a large organization. If we want to organize as a union, we are opposed by the hospitals and other well-financed anti-union forces. Critics of unions have asked us to justify why we need a union. I am amazed at the irony of that question. A hospital does not need to justify itself as an organization, but if a group of nurses want to organize, that is something that needs to be explained.

The reason we face challenges to our solidarity is clear. We as organized nurses can advocate for better wages, better working conditions, and the job protections that would prevent the need for the bullying that I have just described. That means hospitals would need to pay nurses more, and incur more costs in terms of wages, benefits, and overall working conditions. Hospitals would face limitations to their power to make decisions and changes. I understand why hospitals would want to counter my efforts to organize, but that does not mean I am not justified in my actions. As an individual, I have every right to advocate for my interests, just as the hospital administrator does. But the difference is that I am advocating for myself, mostly on my own time and at my own expense.

When we nurses often think of ourselves as professionals, sometimes we conclude that we do not need unions or any other collective organization. This is unfortunate and faulty reasoning. Organizationally, we're more like blue-collar workers. We are a large group that is employed directly by hospitals to perform roughly similar tasks with similar skills.

Cynthia, the nursing manager of a large department in a middle American city hospital I introduced earlier, Explained to me her feelings about unions. Her role at the hospital is typical of nursing management, and she hates unions. It is not a visceral hatred, but she sees them as a threat to her ability to run her department.

She described to me the *Just Culture* policy of the hospital, in which nurses are not punished for mistakes because they are only human. Also, Cynthia would lose good nurses if she were not treating them fairly. To prove her point, she gave me a flow chart titled the *Corrective Action Decision Tree*. If a nurse made a single mistake that was an honest error and not negligent, she faced little or no negative effects. If that nurse was repeatedly making errors or demonstrating reckless behavior, disciplinary measures would follow. This was all the same as I heard from Linda of the North Carolina Nursing Board. Cynthia explained that at her hospital, they respect each other, resolve differences fairly, and can look forward to job security as long as they did their jobs properly. No need for unions here.

So far, so good. As I looked at the documents she provided me, I noticed they referred to patient safety. There was a lot of talk about how nurses need to ensure patient safety. That I have no issue with. But there was no mention of ensuring the nurses' job security. I asked her where I could find that *Just Culture* policy on the hospital's website. It wasn't there, and she couldn't find it on any publicly available document. I contacted the hospital's public affairs office, asking about their *Just Culture* policy. They didn't respond to my repeated calls and emails.

Keeping an open mind, I asked her about work life in her hospital. Cynthia responded that she does not want a union because it is easier for her to just call a nurse in and talk one to one. That's a good deal for

117

Cynthia, but what about the nurse? When it comes to power gradients, those with power often don't see it. She calls a nurse into her office and thinks she is having an open, honest conversation. I would not describe a conversation between a manager and an employee in that manager's office as an open, honest conversation.

Does this hospital have any cliques or mafias? That's when she paused and noted, "Actually, all the Filipinos work on the night shift. It pays better when you work nights." So all the Filipinos are on the night shift, and the night shift consists of all Filipinos. That made me stop in my tracks. She did not have an explanation for why one ethnic group was clumped together and disproportionately working the night shift, except that they wanted the money.

I asked more questions: "Do the nurses feel stressed or burned out?" No, they get breaks, but she added, "Sometimes they refuse the breaks because they're so worried about making a mistake. Some nurses would rather work through breaks because they don't want to make a mistake and get sued or get in trouble with the nursing board." Wait a minute. She just told me the *Just Culture* policy means her nurses won't be penalized for making an honest mistake. Now she's describing how they pass up breaks (which is probably a violation of the law) out of fear of making mistakes.

Cynthia is highly educated, experienced, and sincere about people's welfare. I can say this having known her for a long, long time. But I'm realistic enough to realize we all have our blind spots. She has been a nursing manager for so long, she has, in my view, internalized the hospital's interests as her own. When I pointed out the fact that she was showing me internal hospital documents without authorization, she replied, "that's fine. The hospital is open and fair about these things." I wouldn't be so sure about that.

Another challenge to nurse solidarity has to do with the dynamics of the nursing profession. In other professions, workers enjoy a solidarity because there is an "us against them" mentality. For example, police, and many unionized labor groups, have a tight bond among themselves because they need a united front against a common foe. Nurses do not have this. The "foe" may be the supervisor, the patient, or the hospital. None of these make for good foes to unite nurses. The supervisor is often a fellow nurse who was promoted and who is protecting and maintaining the existing clique. Union rhetoric makes the hospitals out to be the foe against which we need to unite. But often our hospitals, where people come seeking our aid, do not make for a good enemy.

Nursing Organizing for the Common Good

The bullying I described is but one example of how nurses react to their overworked situation. It may not be clear that that is what is happening, or who is bullying whom. As we move our profession toward greater solidarity, the goal is to reduce these negative interactions and build teamwork, instead of pointing fingers and making accusations.

Gina was faced with a near-impossible job situation in which she was forced out and had to seek legal support. She found, with the help of her lawyers, a large pool of other nurses that had also suffered from the policies of that hospital chain. They brought legal action and won. Nurses organize out of necessity. I have some concerns about using this litigious route as the best route forward for solving our problems. First and foremost, this was only done after Gina had lost her job. The goal here is for her to get to continue in the job she loves and with an employer that respects her. Second, it is a horribly expensive way to resolve disputes. Imagine how much extra that hospital paid compared to if they had done the right thing in the first place. Third and most important, this is not an example of nurses organizing among themselves for their common good. After the lawsuit, there was no more organization. They, as a group, were compensated, and then they went their separate ways.

Theresa Puckett had a different experience from Gina, and one that could help managers like Cynthia see the world from a more promising angle. Theresa, based in Ohio, is a rarity because she has a PhD and still works in direct patient care. She recognizes that her credibility as a nurse scholar is based on her close connection to patient care, and that her clinical work is enhanced by her academic training, which few other nurses have. She worked for a local university hospital as a PRN nurse (for *pro re nata* in Latin, meaning "as needed"). Whereas registry nurses work for an agency, a PRN nurse works directly for the hospital, but on an as-needed basis. She was well liked by her fellow nurses and also taught in local nursing programs.

As do many other nurses, she got sick. We work in highly stressful conditions, exposed to every possible infectious agent, and for her to fall ill was not unexpected. She called in sick, knowing that if she were to go

119

to work, the patients would be exposed to her illness and suffer. The hospital has a policy that if a nurse has two or more unexcused absences in 60 days, she can be terminated. Theresa has chills, coughs, dizzy, and a runny nose. She also had a doctor's note saying she should not go to work.

Theresa's manager may not have been unsympathetic to her cause, but remember what I said about hospitals being organizations and managers needing to represent their employer. In this case, her manager wanted to be fair and equitable. The policy was that an employee *may* be fired for two unexcused absence. That gave the manager some discretion. But her manager didn't want to be accused of favoritism, so she fired anyone who met the criteria. Theresa recalls the irony of reading posters on the hospital walls warning people to stay away if they are sick and infectious.

Theresa, being a highly qualified nurse, was not short of work opportunities. What concerned her more than losing this particular job was the effect of this policy on the nursing workforce of that hospital, and the effect it would have on patient safety. Government regulations say a hospital should not allow workers to come to work sick, but it does not require them to stay home. Theresa is now organizing with other nurses to change that rule. They want it to be stronger, so that a hospital is not allowed to have sick nurses working in patient care. She has joined forces with Janie Garner of the organization Show Me Your Stethoscope.

I asked her about the role of unions in Ohio. There are a few unionized nurses, but they are few and far between. There was not much chance of using Theresa's case to organize the nurses as a whole for collective action. Imagine how this story would have played out if unions had much power in that area.

One of the best examples of nurses organizing comes from California based Kaiser Permanente (KP). They are more than just a hospital chain but offer a comprehensive healthcare system for its members. Nursing scholar Suzanne Gordon compared the Veterans Administration to KP, both being examples of what a world-class healthcare system might look like. Another thing they both share is a highly unionized workforce.

Besides being on the cutting edge of healthcare, KP partnered with the labor unions early on to create a system of shared management that continues today as an example of how there does not need to be an antagonistic relationship between individual nurses and their managers, and the unions and the hospitals. When I worked for KP, the managers would simply refuse to meet with me without a union representative present. I actually felt closer and safer to management in those cases because I was on something closer to an even power level with them.

Some of the criticisms I have heard about unions have some merit, which is why nurses need to be sophisticated in how they approach their solidarity. Ideally, unions are stable and have a solid organizational structure of its own. They cannot operate without adequate funding and coherent organization. They get criticized for spending money on administration, yet compared to the hospitals they work with, the overhead is usually quite small. A benefit to being in a well-organized union is accountability. There have been cases of serious abuses by unions, of their power and money. In those cases, it was because there were not the organizational safeguards that come from a well-run organization.

Unions have been known to get involved in political and social issues that have little or nothing to do with their members' interests. For example, in San Francisco, I have seen unions getting involved with rent control and affordable housing. While that is an important issue for many, that does not make it a union issue.

Unions need the active participation of their members. This has proven challenging because nurses are already overworked. Spending time on union matters is something some of us would rather not do if given a choice. We may not think it is important, but it is. By actively involving the members on an ongoing basis, there is a double benefit of increased credibility on the part of the union and a broader and more powerful message being sent to the employers.

But I still would like to avoid the us-against-them situation, which does not move the nursing profession forward. There are direct care nurses like Theresa and myself, as well as the nurse mangers like Cynthia. We are all nurses, and we need to work together. Yet we sit on opposite sides of the union-management table. This is a problem that is going to require the kind of sophisticated solution that healthcare professionals are known for. If we can work our magic in the realm of healthcare, we should also be able to do something comparable in organizing ourselves as nurses.

Chapter 5 References

[1] Sweller, "Cognitive Load During Problem Solving."

[2] Tennant *et al.*, "The Concept of Stress."

[3] Record Research Staff, "Anderson man arrested …"

[4] Menzies, "A Case-Study …"

[5] Aiken *et al.*, "Hospital Nurse Staffing …"

[6] Robertson, " Nurses (still) wanted."

[7] Jameton, *Nursing Practice: The Ethical Decisions.*

[8] Aiken *et al.*, "Implications of the California Nurse Staffing Mandate."

[9] Sochalski, "Nursing Shortage Redux."

[10] Mealer *et al.*, "Increased Prevalence of Post-Traumatic Stress Disorder …"

[11] Burgess *et al.*, " Personality, Stress and Coping in Intensive Care Nurses."

[12] Vessey *et al.*, "Bullying, Harassment, and Horizontal Violence," 136.

[13] Scott *et al.*, "What Do Nurses and Midwives Value About their Jobs?" From a survey done in Victoria, Australia (n=990), 17 percent is a mix of 16 percent for nurses and 19 percent for midwifes, survey.

[14] Jack, *Silencing the Self*; Jack, *Behind the Mask.*

[15] Vessey *et al.*, "Bullying, Harassment, and Horizontal Violence."

[16] See, e.g., Bilgel *et al.*, "Bullying in Turkish White-Collar Workers."

[17] Vessey *et al.*, "Bullying, Harassment, and Horizontal Violence." The authors note that with respect to data on bullying, "research evidence is scant."

[18] Vessey *et al.*, "Bullying, Harassment, and Horizontal Violence," 141.

[19] Thomas, *Transforming Nurses' Anger and Pain*, 106.

[20] Bickel, "Why Do Women Hamper Other Women?"

[21] Vessey *et al.*, "Bullying, Harassment, and Horizontal Violence," 143.

[22] Vessey *et al.*, "Bullying of Staff Registered Nurses in the Workplace," 301.

[23] Vessey *et al.*, "Bullying, Harassment, and Horizontal Violence," 136–140.

[24] Roberts, "Oppressed Group Behavior."

[25] Freire, *Pedagogy of the Oppressed.*

[26] Hutchinson *et al.*, "Workplace Bullying in Nursing."

[27] Vessey *et al.*, "Bullying, Harassment, and Horizontal Violence, "147.

[28] Vessey *et al.*, "Bullying of Staff Registered Nurses in the Workplace," 304.

[29] D'Ambra and Andrews, "Incivility, Retention and New Graduate Nurses."

[30] Brown, *The Shift*. To be clear, the book is not autobiographical. Brown presents an exemplar of the kind of thing that does happen in a hospital, but not what she herself has done.

[31] Curtis *et al.*, "You Have No Credibility.

6

On the Road to State Nursing Boards

In chapter 1, I wrote of my visits to nursing boards around the United States—spurred by my first visit to a board, in California. Here, I want to pick up where chapter 1 left off, and share my observations from travels to state board meetings not mentioned there—beginning with Connecticut, where I visited in February 2016. At the time, it was the longest trip I had made for a nursing board meeting.

The southwest part of Connecticut includes some of the wealthier suburbs of New York City, and the state is home to one of the Ivy League schools, Yale University—which has a nursing school. I had high expectations of this state's nursing board, officially called the Board of Examiners for Nursing. My assumption had always been that states with top-ranked nursing schools would have state nursing boards that perform better than those in other states. Surely one of the nurses at the schools of high repute, I thought, would take an interest in the board and push the board to maintain higher standards.

My Connecticut experience revealed that my bias was unjustified.

The meeting was in a side room of a state office building in a distant corner of Hartford, the state's capitol. The room was dark, there were not nearly enough chairs for the public, and we could not hear much of what was going on. It was as if the board was holding a "public meeting" in name only. After a couple hours, it was over.

The board could have used the occasion to have significant interactions with the public, but instead this gathering simply fulfilled a legal mandate to hold a meeting in which the public could be in the same room—nothing more. Two years later, when I visited Pennsylvania, I encountered something quite similar. The board seemed simply to be fulfilling a legal requirement to hold a public meeting. There, board members sat facing each other at long, U-shaped tables while the public could not see much more than the two members sitting at each table's end. We could not hear most of what was going on, and we couldn't see who was doing the talking.

One thing I did pick up from the Connecticut meeting was a disciplinary case in which a nurse who worked in multiple states had made a complaint about a doctor at one of her job sites. It was an example of how nurses can face disciplinary action for anything, anywhere, at any time. In this particular case, the nurse had spent some time working in Texas, and that's where a complaint had been filed against her. In Connecticut, as in most states, anyone with a disciplinary case in any other state is automatically subject to investigation. Even if that case in the other state has no merit, Connecticut will still make the nurse suffer through an investigation.

Imagine a traveling nurse trying to defend herself from a spurious accusation in a state she no longer works in two thousand miles away. I don't know the details of where this nurse worked or resided, but she found herself reported to the board in Texas for sleeping on the job and being slow to respond. She defended herself, stating she was awake but simply had her eyes closed. Her explanation for this accusation of sleeping on the job was that she was being targeted. When I heard the complaint against her, the first thing I thought was that there was more to the story than we were hearing.

Amazingly, a board member acknowledged the situation the nurse found herself in, having filed her complaint against the doctor. "Once you make a complaint, you're on your own. Nobody has your back." In other words, if you file a complaint against any other person of power, you have a target on your back. It was the essence of what I have observed repeatedly: accusations against a nurse say more about the power structure than about the particular nurse. In a profession where only one in a thousand mistakes gets reported, it's impossible not to wonder what it was about that *one* nurse or that *one* "mistake" that caused it to be the one to be reported, as opposed to any of the others.

Also, notice how a nurse working in multiple states can be forced to defend herself everywhere against an accusation made in a faraway place, because all the other states simply have a knee-jerk reaction to the first accusation. One accusation can put a nurse into bankrupting litigation across the country. Every state that I am aware of has this policy of starting an investigation if any other state starts an investigation. I'm not sure what the alternative is, but the process has the overall effect of creating a lot of work for boards and lawyers while bankrupting the nurse in question and destroying her reputation.

Perhaps the nurse in question at that board meeting was looking for an excuse to explain why she was involved in a disciplinary case. But even so, the board demonstrated that it had at least one member who saw what I had noticed long before but that had never been stated in any other board meeting I'd attended.

After Connecticut, I returned to the Midwest with a trip to the Michigan Board of Nursing in April 2016. My visit played out a lot differently than I expected. I flew to Chicago and then drove to Lansing, the state capital, for an overnight stay in a hotel. The next morning it was snowing, and I walked several blocks through Michigan's massive government office complex to the board's building, only to discover that only the disciplinary committee and not the full board was meeting that day. That committee meeting wasn't for a couple of hours.

Despite the freezing weather outside, the folks in the lobby were hesitant to let me stay and wait. Finally, board staff called down from the upstairs office, saying I could go from the lobby downstairs to the basement cafeteria and then go down the hall to the committee meeting room at the appropriate time—but stating in no uncertain terms that I was forbidden to go anywhere else in the building.

Committees are common to nursing boards; most boards delegate to committees much of the work, particularly disciplinary matters. These committees typically consist of a few board members. The Michigan disciplinary meeting had a few board members, plus a lawyer there to help these board members understand and adhere to the law.

Some boards are stricter than others when it comes to discipline.

Others are more liberal. Some boards give a nurse accused of some wrongdoing the benefit of the doubt. Demetrius Porche, head of Louisiana's nursing board and a prominent leader in the board community, once stated before The American Association of Nurse Attorneys (TAANA) that he would invite a nurse facing discipline to explain what she was thinking. His intention was to give her the chance to show that she had good intentions despite having made a mistake. His statement struck me as a little odd, since his earlier comments at that conference had made him sound condescending to nurses. The liberal approach he described is not an established norm. Some boards, such as the one in Nevada, seem to show no concern with giving nurses the benefit of the doubt. The approach in Michigan seemed much closer to Nevada's than to that of Louisiana.

That snowy morning, Michigan's disciplinary committee was considering the case of a nurse accused of some wrongdoing—exactly what it was went unstated in the meeting—that got her removed from the floor in her hospital. In other words, she was no long taking care of patients that day. From what I could discern, she was called into a meeting with her managers and then left to go home.

The committee was trying to prosecute the nurse, who was not present at the meeting, for "patient abandonment"—a serious offense. The charge seemed to stem from her leaving the hospital; it was not stated whether abandonment was the only accusation or there had been some preceding "wrongdoing" that led the nurse to be reported. The legal counsel told the committee that the nurse could not be accused of patient abandonment because she didn't have any patients at the time she left the hospital.

Board and committee meetings can be tedious, but this was one of those moments when things get interesting—that is, when I get to watch members make important decisions in real time. There were a lot of factors at play. First of all, the committee should not have been deciding the nurse's fate when there hadn't even been an investigation by the board staff, which would have calmly and without the pressure of time been able to think about the best thing to do.

One committee member asked the legal counsel what the nurse *could* be prosecuted for, and the lawyer suggested "unprofessional conduct." It was clear to me that the committee was openly looking for some way, *any* way, to punish the nurse. When you cook spaghetti, sometimes you throw a piece against the wall to see whether it sticks. If it does, the spaghetti's ready to eat. In this case, the committee seemed to be throwing accusations against the wall to see what might stick. I was shocked at this kind of approach to discipline, but I guess my Nevada experience should have prepared me for anything.

In the end, the committee's decision was to move forward with "unprofessional conduct." Later, I called Michigan's board to get some background information about the case, but was told there was no public information available. So I have no idea what the whole case was about other than what I overheard at the meeting. The minutes of the meeting are not a transcript, so no one who was not present at that time could know what was said. The published minutes state that the nurse "will be place [*sic*] on probation for a minimum of one day, not to exceed one year, with continuing education in professional accountability/legal liability and medication errors. Respondent is to pay a $250.00 fine within 90 days."

What also struck me about the meeting was how they could say these things in an open meeting, without any apparent concern that the public was present. It was as if they saw nothing wrong with this spaghetti approach to prosecution. It is not unusual for boards to receive reports of possible wrongdoing, and the board *does* need to determine whether some nursing rule was violated or a crime was committed. But nurses in every state run the risk that once accused of anything, they are then put under a microscope—and all of their actions may be judged and perhaps even prosecuted. The mere fact of being reported to a board can jeopardize a nurse's career, since many nursing employers ask applicants to indicate such actions when applying for jobs.

That Michigan nurse was "only" placed on probation and fined $250, but having *any* disciplinary action on your record is major strike against you. For the rest of her career, if anyone ever has a conflict with her at work, an accusation can be made and the Michigan board's action will be used to show a "pattern" of mistakes.

Michigan was doing what many other states do—looking for a violation to match the nurse's actions, instead of, as Porche suggested, assuming innocence until proven otherwise. In Michigan's case, the main difference was that I and the other public members present could at least witness the process. There were only a couple of other people present, including other nurses there for their own disciplinary hearings. Just as in almost every other board meeting across the country I've attended, no representatives of nursing professional associations and labor unions were present. I can't help but wonder whether board members would be a lot more careful in how they handle these disciplinary cases if they faced the kind of scrutiny of their conduct that would be provided by the organizations that represent us as nurses.

My next trip to a nursing board came that June—to Iowa, right in America's "heartland."

I love maps, but I hate looking at the map on my phone. I love the paper kind. On a paper map, you can get the big picture, and see what an area has to offer. So, after I flew into Des Moines and picked up my rental car, I stopped at the first convenience store I found, across the street from the airport. I bought a map of the capital city.

As I stood in the parking lot next to the car, with the map open, the first person that walked by asked where I was heading and then he gave me directions to my hotel. Great, I thought, and thanked him. Then I waited until he left to open the map again. I really just wanted to peruse the map. Then the next person walking by asked if he could assist with directions.

"Jeez," I thought, "you can't even open up a map in public in this town without someone being helpful." Classic American heartland.

After checking into my hotel, I went downtown to familiarize myself with the nursing board office and where the next day's meeting of the Iowa Board of Nursing would be held. In some states, these meetings are held in the state office building the board is in, but sometimes not. Iowa's was in a conference hotel across town, conveniently next to a hospital where you can watch medevac helicopters landing and taking off from the roof. A sports stadium and the Iowa Events Center were both a few blocks away.

Downtown Des Moines was awash with people. There were lots of teenage girls waiting for that night's Justin Bieber concert at the Event Center, but mixed in with them were lots of elderly couples dressed in these interesting and colorful matching outfits. I wondered what was going on. It turned out that the 65th National Square Dance Convention was taking place just across the street from the Bieber concert. I found myself trying to imagine Justin Bieber with Selena Gomez, his girlfriend at the time, in square dancing outfits.

The helpfulness of the folks in the convenience store parking lot confirmed at least one stereotype of Middle America, but the one about it being dull was absolutely not true.

While everyone in this country is presumed innocent, at least officially, nursing boards tend to afford the accusers of nurse defendants additional weight than the defendants themselves. That any nurse who has been accused of wrongdoing is presumed guilty, though, would be misleading. Rather, the situation is one of what we might call *difficult* defense. This results from the disadvantage of the defendant. She is standing before the board defending herself, while all the other nurses in her state are busy working. The board cannot easily compare the defendant's performance with her nurse coworkers or even the "average" performance of nurses in the state. This naturally creates a strong advantage for accusers.

At the Iowa board meeting, a nurse educator at a nursing home had reported a nurse that worked at the same facility. The defendant wasn't present, but her name was stated. It was an African name. I mention that because it struck me that it might be relevant to how the accuser had come to bring the case before the board. The accuser, I should note, wasn't even in a supervisory capacity, and wasn't reporting the nurse in any official role.

The role played by race in any disagreement can be subtle but important. Iowa's ethnic diversity is nothing close to, say, that of California or New York. For an African, living in a place like Iowa can be quite different than in some other parts of the country.

The accuser made it clear to the board members that her report was personal, and that she simply thought the accused nurse was incompetent. Her accusation boiled down to two things, neither of which were very specific: that the accused could be "defensive" and wasn't a "team player."

The accuser gave an example she thought buttressed her claim. One day, another nurse found a patient of the accused was "not looking well." The accused nurse was in another room at that moment. When the accused came into the patient's room, she did seem—according to the nurse educator standing before the board and making the accusation—appreciative of the other nurse's help, and wanted to take control of the situation. Where, I thought, was there any wrongdoing?

The accuser concluded her example by telling the board, "I just don't think that's a good way to be a nurse."

Sure, I thought, the entire situation was less than ideal, but there was nothing in the testimony that came close to warranting discipline. But I didn't get the impression that the board members saw a problem in the accuser's "best" example of wrongdoing. Instead, board members were nodding in agreement with the accuser.

My impression of the Iowa nursing board was that its members are professional, well organized, and thoughtful. But they also seemed prone to the mistake of giving deference to accusers. I wondered if just as they can't compare the work of a single nurse to all the other nurses, they don't get to see what their work as a board looks like compared to other boards.

I certainly could make comparisons, though—more and more.

In August 2016, I headed out in August 2016 to visit yet another one—the Utah State Board of Nursing, which stands out for its substance abuse diversion program. I have never seen such close contact between the board members and the nurses there to defend themselves.

The Utah nursing board meeting I attended that August was held in a small conference room of a large downtown Salt Lake City office building. We visitors sat along the wall, within arm's reach of the board members. In other states, boards had their rooms set up to keep them more separated from the public. I witnessed a board member at a meeting in another state warn someone from the public who had the audacity to approach the board's space to back up and not step behind the tables.

At first, I thought Utah's physical setup was a good thing; the close proximity of board members with the public was a constant reminder to the board members that they were doing their work in public. It also allowed the public, whether it be nurses defensing themselves in disciplinary cases or visitors such as myself, to speak directly to them. Later, after returning home from the Utah meeting, I had second thoughts. That same closeness can also intimidate a nurse coming before the board for disciplinary cases. She has no space in that room to call her own. She cannot talk to a confidant sitting beside her without everyone in the room hearing what is said. Board members can call for a closed session at any time, but nurses coming to a meeting can only use the crowded, busy, public hallway.

The disciplinary session at this meeting was dominated by cases involving impaired nurses. A woman who was in charge of the board's diversion program presented the cases and made recommendations, which was not unusual. But what was odd was the intimacy between the impaired nurses themselves and this diversion program coordinator. The latter's job was to determine their fitness to work as nurses and recommend, if necessary, that their licenses be taken away. And yet, between cases, the impaired nurses were talking to the coordinator as a counselor and friend. One nurse even gave her a hug and thanked her for all she had done.

Were I that diversion program coordinator, I would make it clear there is a professional line that should not be crossed. Apparently, Utah does not have that line. If your role includes the ability to punish and discipline someone, you should not also be claiming to be, or even pretending to be, that person's friend or confidante. In Utah, the person responsible for figuring out how fit nurses may be to work was acting as if she was their friend. Good for that board staff member to gain such confidence—but it's a trap for the nurse.

Imagine you are accused of a crime. You arrive in court to defend yourself without a lawyer to advise you. Before the proceedings begin, the prosecutor comes over and pretends to be your friend—even asking you personal questions, the answers to which could be held against you, help find you guilty, and ultimately end your career. That was how things seemed to be playing out in the Utah board meeting.

One case that came before the board that day involved a nurse who came before the members on a rolling crutch. She reminded me a bit of the nurse I'd seen a year earlier in New Mexico, who also came in on a rolling crutch. This particular nurse had a history of alcohol use. She showed up with no legal counsel and was representing herself.

Throughout the proceeding, she struggled to keep herself together. At one point, she began to cry. She had been in the state's diversion program and seemed to be doing well, and from what I gathered was on track to getting back to working. But after the board members saw her crying, they said they would "reopen her case." I interpreted that to mean she was going to lose her license for the way she presented herself in that room. She did not understand and thought everything was fine.

When I left the building after the meeting, I happened to see her waiting for the bus. The rolling crutch made it a struggle for her to get around, and so I introduced myself and offered her a ride. I also made it clear that I had been at the meeting only to observe was not affiliated with the board in any way. We chatted in my rental car, and I learned that she was employed at the top university hospital and on her way to work. She was calm and coherent. She told me about all the hiking she had done in the area.

I thought to myself that if only she had spoken to the board the way she was talking to me, or if she had had good representation, her case may have turned out much differently. The board staff member running the diversion program acted like a friend, and this nurse bought it. With her guard down and having the mistaken impression that she was in a safe place, she cried. And she talked. And in so doing, she showed her vulnerable side. But it was not a safe place, and those board members and the diversion program coordinator were not her friends. The state of Utah would go on with or without ending that nurse's career.

I didn't know the answer to whether that nurse was truly unfit, but her case is a good example of the challenge all nurses face. We work in high-pressure environments in which mistakes are constantly happening—some unavoidable, but others that reflect a given nurse's unfitness for the job. The mere *accusation* of having made a mistake or being unfit can put a nurse before the board, which itself can damage one's career.

If a nurse has a problem such as substance abuse, friends and good legal representation can help out. Absent friends or legal representation, a nurse's case can turn out like that nurse in Utah. That is why, I believe, we nurses tend to surround ourselves in our workplaces with those we feel will protect us as friends, and bully those we don't think can be trusted.

A short while after my visit, it came to light publicly that a nurse working in a Salt Lake City hospital emergency department had been arrested by a police officer the previous month after she refused his "order" to take a blood sample from an unconscious patient who had been a victim in a crash. A different cop's body cam video showed the sobbing nurse being handcuffed and dragged out the door to a police car. It went viral, adding to the national debate over excessive force. Ultimately, the cop was demoted; Alex Wubbels, the nurse, later reached a settlement for half a million dollars.

Taking that blood sample would have been illegal. Imagine if there had been no witnesses or no recording of what happened. If something that outrageous could play out in front of a camera, think of what might be going on "behind the scenes." In her case, Alex Wubbels, the nurse, was absolutely in the right. What if things weren't so cut and dry?

Nurses work in high-pressure environments in which lots of other people may have their own agendas, some of which may conflict with the nurse's duties. In my visit to Utah, I saw one nurse who seemed to have a problem with substance abuse and worked in a hospital with its own institutional agenda. Other nurses with whom she worked may have been her friend, or not. Other than members of the board and me—the only outside witness at that day's meeting—almost no one knows of her case. At the same time, countless people came to know what happened to RN Wubbels. Had the video not been shared around the world, she would have been an unknown martyr, a good nurse victimized by a clueless cop.

The lesson: a nurse can be viewed as unfit and even a threat to society, or as a hero and martyr, depending on what the public is allowed to see. This pertains no matter the state—something I saw reinforced time and again as I continued to visit nursing boards. My next one was in Arkansas.

The room in Little Rock was impressive when I visited in September 2016, with a massive mural of the nursing board itself on the wall behind the group seated at the front. The audience for the meeting of the Arkansas State Board of Nursing was different than I'd seen for other boards; this one was obviously made up of people from two nursing schools, all wearing their official clinical uniforms. It was striking that all the students from one school were white, and all the students from the other were black.

I asked someone about that. "One's a private school, and the other's a public school," she answered, as if it was perfectly normal.

The meeting itself was all about hearing disciplinary cases. From my experience at other state boards, I was already of the opinion that the process was unjust. Some of the cases involved "incompetent" nursing by nurses who may not have been properly trained, or who perhaps were not really fit for any nursing job. At board meetings in other states, I had heard board members delve into what the nurse whose case was being heard might have been thinking when the actions in question happened. Their objective always seemed to be to figure out whether the nurse was competent but just in a bad work situation or truly ought to be removed from the profession. At one point, a board member made a refreshingly candid and truthful remark. It was a during a discussion of why some "substandard" nurses hold their positions. When managers are desperate to hire, one board member admitted, "They just need a warm body to fill that position." Never before Arkansas had I encountered a board member suggesting a nurse manager might be at fault for something. That came close to happening at this meeting.

The Arkansas meeting was as close I had ever seen in all my visits to state boards, and in the hospitals where I've worked, a nurse manager genuinely be disciplined. A nurse executive was actually sitting before this board, answering for her conduct—or so I thought. She was the director of nursing at a nursing home, a patient had died, and she had received a letter of reprimand for her conduct. She was before the board to appeal, demanding that the letter be rescinded.

The story was that this nurse manager had prevented the staff from doing CPR on the woman who had died. The patient was full code, so there's no doubt CPR was appropriate at that moment. "It's her time," she had said. "Just let her go."

All she had gotten was a letter of reprimand for that decision, and still she was protesting before the board. The members of the board expressed amazement that she had been treated so lightly. The board president had to remind other members that they were only considering whether to let the letter of reprimand stand. And that's what they did.

My experience—and surely that of other nurses reading this—is that had she been any other nurse *not* in a management position she almost certainly would have lost her license and possibly faced criminal penalties. That this manager should have lost her license over this seemed obvious judging from the facial expressions of board members. Yes, she had been fired from the nursing home, but she was already working at another one as director. In other words, there were no significant consequences for her actions.

When I saw that case on the agenda, I thought I would finally have an example of a board treating a nurse manager by the same standards as any nurse doing patient care. Managers like her have a strong incentive to keep out of direct patient care, but she hadn't done that. Anyone else would have lost her career for what resulted.

After the meeting, I visited Little Rock's famous Central High School, where in September 1957 nine black students had tried to carry out the desegregation of American public schools that had been ordered in the

Supreme Court's *Brown v. Board of Education* three years earlier. Governor Orval Faubus called out the Arkansas National Guard to block their entry; later that month, President Dwight D. Eisenhower sent in federal troops to escort the Little Rock Nine into the school. Today, Central is the only active high school within the boundaries of a U.S. national historical park.

When I entered, I was met by a security guard who looked at me with the expression of "oh, another tourist. It was a school day, with the building full of kids. "Oops," I thought, and left. As I stood outside contemplating what had happened 60 years earlier, an older man walked by, apparently a staff member. We chatted a bit, and I mentioned how nice it was that Central High School is still active. He agreed, but had a look that told me all was not well.

"I wonder if these kids have any appreciation of what they have here," I said. "What others did to make this an integrated school."

"No," he replied. "They mostly don't get it." Then he walked off.

I thought back to the nursing board meeting, with students from two nursing schools in attendance, still separated by race. I was left wondering what local nurses thought about that.

That same month, I visited Ohio. The State of Ohio Board of Nursing has the nicest office of any state board I've visited in the United States—right across the road from the state capitol building, in a luxuriously decorated suite. The board meeting played out like most others, but the disciplinary hearing component had some odd twists. For one, there was no crowd of nursing students, which I've always found to be intimidating to the nurse defendants in these hearings. There would not even have been room for those students—who would have been brought there by their schools only show them kinds of nurses *not* to be.

With only the board and a few others in the room, this venue was more conducive to a respectful hearing rather than a public humiliation. The nursing students of Ohio, I thought, can learn the importance of defending their licenses in other ways—such as having nurses invited to address their classes who had gone through the process.

Or so I thought it was more conducive. The board had a timer it used as defendants gave their defense; it was the loudest, most annoying buzzer I have ever heard. It reminded me of the old TV *Gong Show* from my childhood, where people would come on and perform and if the judges deemed they had no talent, they would bang a huge gong.

The disciplinary hearings were like that: going over the time limit was a major offense met with a deafening noise. After the first victim, all the defendants that followed could see what was coming—and they became the most nervous, shaking, crying defendants I had ever seen.

During the recess, I sat in the lobby next to a well-dressed guy who did not seem familiar with the state board office. He turned out to be a lawyer from a firm representing a man for a drug offense whose wife, a nurse, was defending her license before the board. The lawyer had never done a professional license defense, and had no clue about nursing. His firm had included representing the nurse as an extra for the drug defendant. This is not unusual; in my experience, nurses are always scrounging for legal support that they can afford. The average nurse cannot afford thousands of dollars for a good lawyer when confronted with big problems such as substance abuse or, as in this instance, a spouse in trouble with the law.

Notably, nursing boards know this—but seem not to care in the least. I've not seen a single case in which a board backed off a defendant who showed up without representation and advised her to get good legal advice. Typically, boards view cases involving nurses without legal representation as opportunities to move forward more easily, and are happy they don't have to answer to some formidable, knowledgeable defense attorney.

I see a couple of solutions to this problem. A first step would be for boards to acknowledge that nurses need high-quality legal representation. Nurses should not be seduced into thinking the board is their friend.

I was at a meeting of The American Association of Nurse Attorneys (TAANA) in Savannah, Georgia, when Demetrius Porche, head of Louisiana's nursing board, addressed the audience. TAANA is a nonprofit organization with a membership that includes attorneys and others interested in nursing-related legal issues. Porche spoke of the defendants who come before his board lacking legal representation find themselves ill prepared, overwhelmed, and shocked at the proceedings to which they are being subjected.

"We're not here to enjoy tea and crumpets," he said—stating as a joke a common misperception among nurses of how proceedings might unfold. It's a misperception that leads to exploitation of defendants that show up without representation.

If we want to ensure our nurses have the protection and quality representation they deserve, I would look to unions and professional associations as key. But while nurses' unions already defend some of their members' interests, they do not seem to be playing a proactive role by overseeing board operations. The same goes for our professional associations. While I often see representatives of the associations at portions of meetings that directly affect them, they don't stick around for the disciplinary hearings. In fact, I do not recall ever seeing any union representative at any of disciplinary hearings at any board meeting I've attended, in any state. And while professional associations such as the American Nursing Association are involved in myriad activities, in most states I have visited they do not seem to get involved with boards much at all. I've seen precious little presence of our professional associations at meetings I've attended.

My concern is not the absence of union and association representatives not sitting in on these meetings. Our profession should be controlled by nurses. Our scope of practice and the standards of conduct should be decided in our unions and professional associations, and not by the boards. The boards are filling a vacuum that should not exist, and thus driving our profession—not always to our best interest.

Nurses' unions do take care of many specific needs, such as negotiating salaries and working conditions. They also seem to get involved in political advocacy, including lots of issues that do not directly affect nurses *as nurses*. For example, in the 2018 California statewide election, my state unions were actively supporting a ballot measure to increase rent control. Whether you are for or against rent control, I think we can agree that while it may affect nurses it is not a *nursing* issue *per se*. I met with a New York labor organizer in Albany who described to me his view that unions need to engage in a broad social movement. I could not disagree more. Some nurses are tenants, some are homeowners, and some are landlords. No nurses union or association can, in my opinion, have much of a positive impact when it strays far from what nurses are concerned with *as nurses*. But were unions to get involved with nursing boards, I believe they could have more of an impact for their members. It's a lesson culled from experience after experience at board meetings with unions essentially absent.

I visited Minnesota in October 2016 with high expectations: the members of the Minnesota Board of Nursing publish often on regulatory issues in professional journals, and they seem to be exceptionally active in National Council of State Boards of Nursing activities. It was no surprise, therefore, when in August 2017 the Minnesota board won the NCSBN's Regulatory Achievement Award, recognition for its "identifiable, significant contribution to the mission and vision of NCSBN in promoting public policy related to the safe and effective practice of nursing in the interest of public welfare."*

The board meeting room I entered was different from any other I'd been in. Board members sat at a square table, which the public sat around. This setup removed the typical physical separation I'd seen elsewhere, which isolated board members from the public. Here, they could not avoid interacting with the public even if they tried.

Introductions were made around the room—which was not unusual. Boards in many states begin their meetings by introducing themselves and then asking audience members (when those audiences are very small) to do the same. There were only a few visitors at this Minnesota meeting, and the introductions process made it easy to know who they were and why they were there. One person in the audience was a nursing student who had come on her own initiative—not with a group from her school—just to see what a board meeting was all about. It was one of only two times I ever encountered directly a nurse coming to a board in an individual capacity to see what goes on at a meeting (the other was a curious nurse in Nebraska). There may have been some in other states, but with 300-plus attendees in New Mexico, for instance, how could anyone really know?

I mentioned earlier that the layout of Utah's board meeting was intimate, and that that was a bad thing. In Minnesota, closeness was a good thing. What's the difference? The Utah board was holding its disciplinary hearings in a room that gave defendants no privacy and no sense of personal space. Minnesota was not holding disciplinary hearing in this room, so the closeness was, in my opinion, something positive.

The Minnesota board handled the food issue quite well. As I mentioned about my visit to Washington State, some boards put out food only for members and tell the audience it's not welcome to it. The Nevada board, with hundreds of visitors in the audience, ate in a separate space—so there was no sense of excluding the public. Even in states with only a few visitors, though, boards seem to feel it's okay to lay out their food in front of audience members and then exclude the public. In most of these cases I observed, I was actually the only visitor in the room who was visiting, and thus the only one excluded—which seemed particularly rude.

Minnesota joined the ranks of Nebraska and West Virginia—two states I'd already visited—in not making that mistake and understanding what I consider a simple courtesy. Perhaps the board was not *legally* supposed to let me and the few others share in the food, but we ate. I know there are far more important issues at hand, but I took note of this Minnesota hospitality.

The meeting itself was well organized, with an ambitious agenda that covered a lot of issues. The board members moved through that agenda expeditiously. They had a clear sense of what needed discussion and what could be delegated to committees. I never got the sense that they were wasting time on details.

Among the particulars, the accounting director led board members in a discussion of fiscal responsibility, which told me they took such matters seriously. There was also a discussion on how to orient new board members. When I visited the Colorado board more than a year later and watched as one board member explained to a new member how things worked, I thought back to how Minnesota's focus on a real orientation seemed to get it right.

It was clear to me that this was a state board that placed a high priority on the quality of its meetings, and wasn't just fulfilling a legal mandate to convene. This sense was confirmed when the board ended the meeting with a "Value Reflection." The theme that day was "integrity," and members were asked to cite examples of what they had done recently in their board work that reflected integrity.

I have been thinking long and hard about what goes into the "ideal" nursing board meeting. Minnesota was a good example of a board that does things right. Its website is informative, my phone calls to their office were answered politely, and in every contact I had with the board and staff the information they provided was accurate. Board members take their role seriously and appear to be forward thinking, coming up with ways to work better in the future. A nursing board, though, needs not only to do things right, but also to do the right thing. A board must recognize that it exists not to promote or protect nurses or the nursing profession, but to ensure public safety. Unfortunately, in my visits to meetings around the country, I have seen so many examples of boards getting involved in issues that promote nursing instead of focusing on their core purpose.

To be fair, the typical state board in the United States does a far better job than the national boards in most other countries I've visited. Our overall system of regulating nurses is far more developed and more professional. At least we have actual boards that hold actual meetings; often, other countries have nothing more than websites with information. And where American state boards perform most of the major duties such as issuing licenses, setting performance standards, and disciplining nurses that do not meet those standards, most other countries do not come close.

After a hiatus of many months, I commenced visiting state nursing boards again in June 2017, beginning with Wisconsin. It was an opportunity to observe how a board dealt with one of the biggest issues in nursing regulation across the United States, and a major topic for boards—the Nurse Licensure Compact (NLC). The National Council of State Boards of Nursing (NCSBN) describes the NLC as "increase[ing] access to care while maintaining public protection at the state level."[2] Essentially, it is a legal agreement by states that sign on to recognize the nursing licenses of other states. A nurse with an RN license in one state that is a compact member can work in any of the other states that are compact members.

As of this writing, twenty-nine states are NLC states, and several other states are close to joining. Boards generally like the idea of the compact because it allows their nurses the chance to work in other states with less hassle. For traveling nurses who move around a lot, the NLC is great. It allows them to work in any of the member states without getting additional licenses.

When I attended a Wisconsin Board of Nursing meeting in June 2017, the state had not yet signed on to the NLC. An expert from the NCSBN headquarters was there to give a presentation on the compact and answer questions from board members—who found the NLC complex and were struggling to keep up with the details. One thing the expert mentioned was that labor unions don't like the NLC. Asked why by a board member, he said it had something to do with competition from nurses in other states pushing wages down. But the expert did not elaborate or cite anything specifically stated by any union. He just left it at that.

The main complaint nurse unions have against the compact is that it may create downward pressure on wages. Every spring, the U.S. Bureau of Labor Statistics releases its annual Occupational Employment Statistics Report showing average wages for workers in a variety of sectors, broken down by state.[3] The 2018 report showed average salaries for RNs in the previous year, and ranked the fifty states and the District of Columbia. To illustrate how this downward pressure might work, consider two states—Nevada and Utah. According to the report, an RN in Nevada (ranked #7) made $84,980, on average, in 2017—an average hourly rate of $40.86. In the state next door, Utah (ranked #38), an RN made $63,050—and average hourly rate of $30.31. In other words, a Utah nurse is used to making about 25 percent less than a nurse in next-door Nevada.

Traveling from Utah to Nevada would be relative easy for a nurse interested in working in both states. Imagine RNs at a hospital in Nevada being called in by management and told that all future openings, and all available overtime, will be filled by nurses traveling from Utah—who are going to work for a lower wage, even one midway between the prevailing Nevada hourly rate and the Utah rate. That represents a lower cost for the hospital, a higher wage for the Utah RNs, and downward pressure on the Nevada RNs, who have to wonder whether keeping their local jobs is going to require committing to a wage cut. (And just in case you think the wage differential is a supply-and-demand issue, Utah and Nevada have nearly the same populations and the same number of RNs).

I was dismayed to hear the NCSBN representative, who was there to sell Wisconsin on joining the compact, bring up unions in a negative way and without elaboration. As the expert spoke, I realized that unions have been almost silent on the matter of nursing compacts. If you search the Internet, you'll find a few statements by unions against the compact. That's all.

I already mentioned my disappointment in unions when it comes to their participation in board meetings. Only once have I attended a board meeting and knew of union representatives present, and that was in California. Even there, in a state with one of the strongest nurse unions in the country, union presence at board meetings is sparse. Yet at many of the board meetings I attended, the compact was a major issue of discussion. If the unions oppose the compact, the unions are not doing a good job of getting the word out, and boards seem dismissive of union concerns because they don't even mention this conflict (with the exception of this Wisconsin meeting).

Wisconsin, by the way, adopted the NLC and it became law in the state in January 2018. That was the same month I visited Arizona.

Few nursing board presidents have done what the president of the Arizona State Board of Nursing did at the meeting I attended. He spoke to the nursing students present, explaining how board meetings play out and why the meetings are important to them as soon-to-be nurses. "Our job," he said, "is to make sure every nurse is the best nurse they can be."

Arizona's nursing board deserves credit for trying to make that meeting educational for those nursing students present. I had been encouraged when the board president began talking to the students, but that last statement dismayed me. He was just wrong. It's not the job of nursing boards to make every nurse the best she can be. The job of nursing boards is something very different: to *protect the public* from nurses, when necessary. Removing a bad nurse from the profession may be bad for her as an individual, but it's good for the public.

Some might argue that there is a nursing shortage, and that a nursing board that's doing its job still ought to weigh the benefits of losing a nurse against the cost to society of having one less nurse. But again, these boards have one job: make sure nurses meet a minimum standard, and protect the public from those that do not. That's all.

The Arizona board president made his vexing comment during the morning session. In the afternoon session, the room was full of different students. He gave the same background talk, and I waited for him to end with the "our job" statement he had made that morning. He did not. In the afternoon, he got it right: that boards protect the public and not necessarily the nurse.

The president wasn't the only board member to speak directly to the students. Another board member posed a question to them with the aim of what seemed to be teaching a lesson. "Can you post on social media that you are a nurse and had a bad day?" the board member asked. She then answered her own question: "Keep your professional life professional and your personal life personal."

I could see how difficult it could be to serve the students' interests. The board needed to provide a carefully crafted message on complex matters, but the comment about using social media was totally unrealistic. One of the hallmarks of our profession is that we *do* need to take this personally.

I thought about Jean Watson. Even though I disagree with a lot of her positions on caring, she is right that a good nurse cannot and should not have a wall between her work life and her personal life. Nurses need to be more involved with the profession, advocating for better health policy, and using their skills whenever the need arises. Sometimes, that means going over that wall. When I met her for breakfast in her home town, she was gracious and welcoming, and we had a long talk about nursing and caring. Here was one of the most famous nurses in the world, allowing me take up her time without agenda or ulterior motive.

On more than one occasion, when on a commercial airline, I have responded to requests for medical personnel on board to help with emergencies. Some nurses have told me that when they are on a plane and the flight attendant asks whether there are any medical professionals available to help, they stay as quiet as other passengers. They simply stay put, as if just another passenger.

I see two issues there. The first is whether you should let your personal feelings affect your relationship with patients. On that point, I disagree with Watson. I don't think nurses should bring their personal feelings to work; we should keep our personal and work lives separate. My patient care does not depend in the slightest about how I feel about any type of individual or any group, such as immigrants, the wealthy, and so on. The other is whether a nurse steps up whenever the need arises, such as in a medical emergency situation on the plane. In that case, I absolutely demand a nurse comes forward and help. For a nurse to stand idly by in a medical emergency, when help is needed, would be like an armed, off-duty cop watching a person get mugged and doing nothing.

Had that board member been challenged on her comment, I'm sure she would have provided some nuance. But the mere fact that she could make such an unrealistic statement to a group of students is an example of the kinds of contradictions we work with every day as nurses.

I visited three other states in January 2018 in different parts of the country. One was Colorado. The natural beauty of the Rockies and Denver's mix of world-class urban life mixed with middle-American ranch and agricultural life makes it one of my favorite states to visit.

The Colorado Board of Nursing meeting I attended took place in a high-rise office building in the heart of downtown Denver, in a room about four times larger than what was needed. It was an odd contrast to the meetings I've attended in many other states that jam everyone into small rooms.

That meeting was also the first meeting of a new board member. Another board member took time, as part of the meeting, to explain publicly to her how things worked. By this time, I had been at enough meetings of other boards to know what was about to happen: a board member showing up without any real preparation was going to be voting on issues that could profoundly affect the state's healthcare system or the career of individual nurses who appear before the board.

It reminded me of my visit to Nevada's board, when one of the LPN members was also new. There were votes that day on important issues, and some of those votes were split. That meant the outcome hinged on one member who was making his decisions without having any board experience. Sure, every board at one time or another will have to deal with new members, but some states seem to make the lack of preparation more obvious than others.

Colorado's board, like most others, spent some time reviewing the NCLEX pass rates of nursing schools. One school had a pass rate of 83 percent; a board member told the school's representative, "I want to see you at 100 percent"—which was followed by an admonition: "Testing. Testing. Testing." It was the same with every board: higher test scores were equated with being safer nurses.

But whether passing the NCLEX tells us whether an applicant is going to be a safe nurse is an open question. I know of no research that has attempted to match NCLEX scores with nursing performance. When I asked Doyoung Kim, the NCSBN senior psychometrician responsible for NCLEX development and testing, whether there had ever been a test of the outcomes, he replied that such research project would be impossible because the data are property of each state.[4] The fact is that while the NCLEX exam itself is the property of the NCSBN, the results—including applicant demographic information and test scores—are owned by each state board. That's the case even if the applicant who takes the exam in one state came from elsewhere and plans to apply for a license in another state.

Kim's answer notwithstanding, though, there's no insurmountable obstacle preventing a state from providing data for research purposes. A researcher would need to determine what measure of performance to use, which raises how to define nursing knowledge and recognize it when it is being demonstrated, as well as what constitutes "competency."

Research of that sort could be among the most valuable of any ever done about nursing, because it would have to include a concerted effort to identify all the current practices currently of thousands of nurses nationwide, which would constitute a consensus of nursing practice.

I guess, though, that's for another time. Back to the Colorado meeting.

Sometimes, a board gets into a deep discussion of issues related to nursing that help them solve a general class of problems but that are not directly related to any case before the board at that moment. When I've witnessed such discussions, they provide a glimpse into how the individual board members think. My first encounter with this had been in Oregon, where the board convened a special meeting the evening before the regular meeting to have just such a discussion. This happened in Colorado, too, although not in a special meeting.

The Colorado board's discussion—which was strictly hypothetical—was about patient abandonment. A scenario was offered: a triage nurse steps away from the desk when there is no patient there. If one is a triage nurse and does not have a patient at that moment, does walking away constitute abandonment? It was an interesting question.

The nurses on the board thought not, but the board's public member was very strict, and said it was like abandoning the patient. That the public member took the hardest line was no surprise to me; I had encountered a couple of other cases in which public members seemed to take very tough stances against nurses. It was yet another case of someone sitting on a nursing board who had thought about an issue a lot more than the average person and who in this instance pushed for the strictest interpretation of patient abandonment. Of course, he had never worked as a nurse.

That discussion in Colorado reinforces an argument I've been making throughout this book: nurses are held to unrealistically high standards.

I visited the Delaware Board of Nursing the same month as Colorado, and there a public member wanted to discipline a nurse that had been involved in a patient death. When the nurse arrived to find an apparently unresponsive patient, the investigation report into the case stated she had seemed slow and not very knowledgeable regarding how to handle a code. Many minutes went by before the paramedics arrived and began CPR. Minutes later, the patient was declared dead.

To that public member of Delaware's board, all that mattered was that the patient had died. He seemed fundamentally unknowledgeable about what nurses face every day. We do not deal with people because they are well. Typically, there is a problem, and sometimes people are at that edge between life and death. That is where the nurse matters most. It puts us in difficult situations and sometimes we are blamed for bad outcomes (deaths).

The nurse members of the Delaware board told the public member that while they thought the nurse's performance had perhaps been subpar, it was not so bad to justify her losing her license and ending her career. What struck me is that they used their personal reputations to make that point. There was no evidence provided on what qualifies as an acceptable standard of care. The nurse members did not cite statistics or scientific proofs. They simply gave their personal judgment. The public member relented.

To be fair, public members of nursing boards are not always stricter than their nurse counterparts. There was the California businessman on that state's board who was the only one protesting that nurses were being filmed in their disciplinary hearings. In Vermont, where I also visited in January 2018, the issue was not so much that the public member of the Vermont State Nursing Board was stricter or more lenient than the nurse members, but simply that he seemed to have no opinion at all, at least as far as I could discern. He served on three Vermont state boards dealing with completely disparate professions, and did not seem to have much of a grasp of anything going on in the nursing board meeting. He just went along with the majority.

When public members take a hardline stance, it reminds me of the members of our community that insist we need to be held to the "highest standards" without thinking through the implications for nurses or patients.

In June 2018, I made my way to Kansas, which like Iowa (where I had visited two years earlier) is considered classic middle America, part of the "heartland." I wondered how the Kansas State Board of Nursing might differ from other boards I'd visited, particularly those in coastal states.

The meeting took place in the state's capitol city, Topeka. It's a small city that houses the Evel Knievel Museum that celebrates the life of one of America's most famous daredevils; and the notorious Westboro Baptist Church, perhaps best known for its public demonstrations at the funerals of fallen servicemen and servicewomen using inflammatory hate speech against LGBTQ people and others. It is also the location of the *Brown v. Board of Education* National Historical Site, which commemorates the legacy of the U.S. Supreme Court's ruling that ended legal segregation in the nation's public schools.

The meeting of the Kansas State Board of Nursing was to take place over two days. On the first morning, I went to the board's office—where, in the lobby, there is a poster about the board's history that notes that the first male nurses were licensed a year after the board was first formed, nearly a century ago. I was ushered into a crowded meeting room within the administrative offices. Within minutes of my arrival, the board voted to go into executive session and I had to leave the room. Executive sessions—held to discuss private matters without public scrutiny—are standard practice for most boards. The public never knows for certain what happens in these closed-door sessions: despite policies on what should discussed in private and what should be public, once there's a private session there's no real way of knowing whether the privacy was justified.

Later that first day, the meeting continued in public session, this time in larger room.

What played out over my two days with the Kansas board was a good example of disorganization and a lack of strategy. No one seemed to be in charge, and there seemed to be little regard for whether the meeting was a good use of what precious little time is set aside for board meetings. For the entire state of Kansas, it should be noted, the nursing profession's regulatory body takes only a few hours every three months to provide the public with a view into what is going on.

At one point, the board spent 15 minutes of that time talking about whether a new printer was needed in the office. Apparently the paper used to print some documents was extra thick, and so is extra hard on the poor existing printer. In the discussion, budgetary issues were raised, as was the question of whether a printer is expensive enough to qualify as a capital asset or is simply an office supply—and so on and so on. I learned more about a particular printer in the Kansas nursing board's office that day than anything about any substantive policy in the state.

It's difficult to pinpoint just how the Kansas board fell into its disorganized process. As in most states I've visited, the session devoted to nursing school regulation was well attended. I thought it a shame that all the nursing school deans left the room as soon as their school as no longer the topic of discussion—not thinking that anything else going on with the board was worth listening to. I'd seen that same thing in state after state.

One nurse in the audience did stick around for me to chat with—and ended up giving me a hint about how things came to be with the Kansas board. She confided, when no one else was within hearing distance, that the previous board executive director was a tyrant who did not allow much room for board members or board staff to contribute to the decision making process. The new executive director, she told me, was improving how the board operates. The decision making process had become more democratic and there was more emphasis on building consensus among board members.

At other state board meetings, I have always held back on sharing my thoughts with people I meet. It's part of my observation method: don't discuss my own impressions or judgments because doing so could affect what people—board members and members of the public alike—might tell me. This time, I broke my own rule and shared with her my impression of the meeting as rather disorganized.

She responded by telling me it used to be a lot worse, and that even things were a little disorganized, at least it was more democratic.

This confirmed my impression from my visits to so many states that the executive director of nearly every board is the kingmaker. She is the one that wields power, even if the public does not see it. Even in California, where there are many high-profile Board members, the executive director is the one that sets the stage and decides much of what is discussed. Board members are not full time. They come together, at most once a month, and in some states for only a couple of full meetings a year. After the meetings, they return to their day jobs. Meanwhile, the board's staff—including the executive director—are together all day, every day, running the program.

Despite a few negatives, I also saw at the meeting one of the most encouraging examples of nursing professionalism. Michelle Knowles, a nurse practitioner working in Hays, was there to be heard. Knowles is a key player in the NP community and active in the NP professional association.

I had to look hard to find Hays on a map. Talk about isolated. But Kansas is a very rural state, and a large number of nurses work in small, isolated communities. They have to work with a lot of independence; they also struggle with a lack of opportunities for learning and growth. As in every other state, nurse practitioners in Kansas are pushing for the right to operate more independently of doctors—but Kansas's law states that NPs only need a doctor to sign off on medications. The board interpreted that law to require a doctor to sign off on *all* NP actions.

This was yet another example of the ongoing tug of war between doctors and nurses over the nursing scope of practice. It is not an easy task, and legal battles usually play out state by state: just because something is allowed in Missouri, for example, it doesn't mean it applies to neighboring Kansas. Nurses end up having to fight the same battle over and over for every little expansion of what we are allowed to do.

Michelle's role with the NP professional association is purely voluntary. On her own time, Michelle drove many hours to attend the meeting and then had to drive all the way back. She had come to point out to the board members what the law actually said and get the board to correct its policy.

This interaction was profound. Among the most important lessons I've learned from visiting these boards is that we nurses need to control our profession. The nursing boards don't represent us; representation comes from professional associations and people like Michelle.

I mentioned earlier how sophisticated and professional the boards in Oregon and Texas are, and how much Texas in particular surprised me. With that in mind, let me continue my travelogue with New York.

Among the most populous states in the country, New York is home to one of the world's largest commercial centers and the United Nations headquarters. Surely the New York State Board of Nursing would rise to the level of Oregon and Texas. But the opposite is true.

A nursing board's website is the main way the outside world can see into the board. It is the best means by which a board can provide information for nurses and the public. To be sure, not all state board websites are the same, and some are better than others. But when it comes to New York State, what is lacking is in a class of its own.

First, the website for nursing doesn't really seem to be the website of the board. I don't think such a website exists. Instead, what does exist is a site maintained by the New York State Office of the Professions (which is responsible for all 36 licensed professions in the state, from acupuncture to land surveying to perfusion and veterinary medicine).

And beyond information about applying for a nursing license, there is almost no other information available.

Over many months, I repeatedly phoned the New York State board to ask about public meetings. I was never able to get any information. So, through a contact at another state's nursing board office, I managed to get the name and email address of the executive director of the New York board. I sent her a message, asking simply whether there would be a public meeting and whether I could meet her some time when I would be in Albany. I also mentioned that the website did not include her name.

The response I received was remarkable. She told me her name was, in fact, on the website. She said absolutely nothing in response to my requests.

I decided to do some detective work. I did a Web search of her name and found the page to which she was probably referring. I am certain that no one would be able to find that page unless they already knew the director's name.

Ever since then, as I continued my travels to board meetings throughout the United States and in other countries, I've kept an eye out for any information about the New York State Board of Nursing. I continue to wonder: Is my impression of this board wrong, or is it just not very good at public relations?

As of this writing, the board seems to remain in hiding, not offering itself to the public and and not taking phone calls.

My last board meeting was in Pennsylvania, in July of 2018. I was starting to see common themes emerge at these meetings, as well as interesting differences. Pennsylvania's meeting room was set up, I hope unintentionally, to discourage public interaction. I sat stuffed between a lot of people in power suits. The board members sat at tables that were perpendicular to our view, so I could only see the side of the person at the end of the table. Audience members were asked to introduce themselves; almost all of them were lawyers. After the board members dealt with a few brief disciplinary cases and some administrative issues, the meeting was over and they quickly left the room.

I felt as if my tour of state board meetings had come to an end, at least for now. Rather than spend more time studying nursing in the United States, I needed to shift gears and focus my attention on other countries.

Chapter 6 References

[*] National Council of State Boards of Nursing, "NCSBN Award Ceremony."

[2] National Council of State Boards of Nursing, "Nurse Licensure Compact."

[3] Nurse.org, "Highest Paying States for Registered Nurses."

[4] Personal communication with the author.

7

Globetrotting

Nurses from other countries are found in hospitals throughout the United States. Sometimes, it may seem as if the majority of nurses in a given hospital are from another country. Some of these nurses were trained elsewhere, and some attended U.S. nursing schools. When they're working in U.S. hospitals, they obviously face the same issues I've discussed in the preceding chapters.

My visits to nursing boards across the United States taught me a lot and helped me get a better understanding of how my country treats nurses and how we regulate nursing, but I came to realize something was missing. So I came up with a perfect quasi-experiment: compare nursing regulations in other countries with those in the United States by visiting those other countries and doing my best to engage nursing leaders in conversations.

That became a sort of "globetrotting"—with the sorts of experiences not specifically about nursing one might expect. The report on my "experiment" in this chapter is thus more story-driven than preceding chapters, in which vignettes served only to illustrate key points.

It was on a trip in February 2017 to several southern African nations that I began visiting nurses and nursing boards in other countries. I wanted a fuller, global picture of nursing's professional landscape. I found a way to give vacations a dual purpose, and began to add visits to nursing educators, regulators, and associations wherever I might be in the world. Eventually, I made some trips specifically for research.

I had visited African several times, all before my mid-career transition to nursing. It was apparent to me that healthcare professionals face different challenges there than in the developed world. This trip was my first time returning to Africa since becoming a nurse, so I was now looking at things differently.

Compared to visiting nursing boards in the United States, I realized I would need an entirely different process. First, I would look online to see whether there were public meetings of some kind of board. It turned out that there were no such meetings in any of the countries I've visited thus far. Without any public meetings to show up at, I took as a next step to email the government's nursing authorities and the country's nursing association.

The southern Africa trip had been planned as a driving tour. It began in the nation of South Africa, which ended apartheid in the early 1990s. In the intervening years, the country has transformed, but at present the government is engaged in a struggle with corruption and crime. In the middle of my first night there, I was awakened by gunfire just outside my hotel. I waited for the sound of police car sirens, but there was no swarm of police. Nothing but quiet. So I rolled over and went back to sleep.

My emails to the government and nursing groups in these African countries had yielded no responses, except in Botswana—where I already had contacts. In hindsight, I should have tried again to make contacts in the other countries once I arrived in Africa, but I did not. So the driving tour ended up being devoid of as much nursing-specific activity as I might otherwise have been able to arrange. I drove from South Africa to Mozambique and then to Swaziland, Lesotho, and back through South Africa to Botswana before returning to Johannesburg.

Swaziland is a landlocked country nearly completely surrounded by South Africa except for its partial border with Mozambique; it is home to a little over 1 million people. Lesotho, with a population of about 2 million, is actually an enclave completely within the borders of South Africa. As I walked the streets of Maseru, Lesotho's capital, and Mbabane, the executive capital of Swaziland, I recalled that HIV rates here hover around 25 percent. The thought kept coming into my mind that one in every four of the people around me was living with HIV.

The next stop on my driving tour was Botswana, north of South

Africa. It's more than five times the area of Lesotho and Swaziland combined, but has only 2.25 million people—meaning there is a lot more open space. I went to the capital city of Gaborone. The dean of the nursing school there, which is part of the national university, earned her PhD from my *alma mater*, UCSF, and I used that as my calling card. She offered a tour of the facility.

The middle of the campus, across from the university library, features a statue of a cow. I asked about it, and learned that it commemorated the campaign to raise money for a national university after the country became independent.

In the 1970s, Botswana—which won its independence from Britain in 1966—was struggling to get the University of Botswana going fully. One of the world's poorest nations at the time, the country began what it called the "One Man, One Beast" campaign, which asked every family in Botswana to contribute grain, eggs, cash, or whatever it could—including a cow that could be auctioned off for cash—to help. It took until 1982, but the university was finally established.

One thing confirmed by this trip was that if I was going to look into nursing in other countries I was going to have to adjust my expectations. I had already heard a lot from African nurses working in the United States about the challenges nurses face in their home countries, which are quite different from those in the United States. I suspected that would be the same situation in many other places I might go. Government regulators don't operate in the same way, and public access to public officials may well be quite different. I would need to put myself out there and try to contact them, which I resolved to do.

My next trip was to New Zealand, in September 2017. The capital city, Wellington, has the most miserable weather of any city I've been to. The good news is that people don't need to worry about their hair—it's pointless. Ever day, it's gale force winds and pouring rain—a stark contrast to the New Zealanders with whom I came in contact, who are among the friendliest I've ever met.

I was running late before my first meeting. Minutes before it was scheduled to begin, I was busily changing into a suit. Then I ran into an office supply store to buy a folio.

My schedule called for meeting with the Nursing Council of New Zealand (the board) that day. I had done my preparation for the council, but once in the lobby of the building, I realized I had mixed up my meetings and locations. Time to improvise.

So, I met first with Jane MacGeorge of the New Zealand Nurses Organisation (NZNO), one of the oldest such associations in the world, tracing its origins all the way back to 1905 when a group of nurses formed the Wellington Private Nurses Association. To put that history in perspective, consider that Florence Nightingale was still alive, nursing professionalism was just forming, and the International Council of Nurses (ICN) was only a year old. When the NZNO joined the ICN seven years later, it was only the eighth national organization to do so.

New Zealand has long been ahead of its time; for instance, in 1893 it became it was the first nation in the world to give women the right to vote, and a year later, the country again made history by requiring compulsory arbitration between employers and unions.

Today, NZNO is the professional association that represents nurses, midwives, and other caregivers. It is also the nation's largest labor union. MacGeorge is the manager of nursing and professional services.

I found it odd that the professional association is also the labor union. She noted that this practice was adopted from the British regulatory system. It is a good example of the sorts of things I learn from visiting boards.

From my perspective, combining a professional association and a union into one organization is a big deal, but not, apparently, to New Zealanders or the British. When I asked MacGeorge about this, she said NZNO sees no conflict between the two roles. I'm skeptical. The job of representing nurses in negotiations over wages and work conditions is fundamentally different from the things a professional association does or ought to be doing—at least to me. When I mentioned that specific concern, she stated that it's just the way things are and there have been no complaints. Besides, they are too busy and underfunded, to worry about what to them is not a pressing issue.

Since then, I've searched for some research into the effects of such a combination, but I've not found any.

As MacGeorge spoke about the cooperation between her organization, the nursing council, and the hospitals, she kept saying what sounded to me like "xia"—until I finally figured out it was her accent and that she was saying "share." NZNO members would share ideas on how best to improve nursing and share opinions with the hospitals and the council. When I meet nurses around the world, I realize that much

156

of my energy is spent simply understanding the words, the English, or the syntax. Only then can I think about what I'm learning about the issues or problems they are facing.

A few days later, I met with the nursing council. The office building that housed the council was directly across from the parking area I used, which wouldn't normally be a problem—but again, I was traveling fast and hard, and logistics were awkward. I was using the car as a changing room, and I had to find a space that ensured no one I might be meeting with could see what I was up to.

That day, the newspaper headline was about a nurse that had been forced to work overtime, leaving her exhausted and fed up. It came in the midst of negotiations for a new contract for nurses in New Zealand. The article itself was about how nurses across the country were being overworked and underpaid.

In my meeting with the council's executive director, I mentioned the headline. The NZNO was in contract negotiations, and this executive director brushed off the article as a ploy by the nurses. When a union contract is due to end and needs to be renegotiated, I have seen various both employers and unions employ various methods as they try to gain an advantage. Sometimes, these include appeals for public sympathy. The union had managed to publicize the plight of one of its nurses and get the local paper to put it on the front page in a very sympathetic light.

The role of the New Zealand nursing council was not clear to me in a situation when nurses were negotiating with their employer, which in New Zealand is the government. A nursing council is supposed to advocate for patient safety, and not necessarily for the needs of nurses. In this case, the combined nursing union–professional association, the NZNO, was making the case that working conditions were jeopardizing patient safety. To me, that would suggest the council had obligation to get involved to ensure nurses were not being overworked. That would be a way I could conceive a nursing council could get involved in union contract negotiations. But it's unheard of in the United States: I have not encountered a single instance in which any U.S. board involved itself in any union contract.

My visits to U.S. nursing boards had begun to give me a good idea of how they should operate and how they should work with professional associations and unions. New Zealand's system is quite different, but most of the issues are the same. Whatever the system, nurses still need to have strong representation from their associations and their unions. The question remains for me of whether one organization can provide both types of representation. That no one in New Zealand seemed to question the arrangement told me that both the NZNO and the nursing council are either ignoring an important issue—which I find unlikely— or that they are, as in most countries, overwhelmed by all the issues affecting nurses.

In February 2018, I took a trip to the Maldives, a country partially on the equator comprised of a chain of 26 atolls with 1,190 coral islands in the deep Indian Ocean, about 620 miles southwest of the southern tip of India. I'm a diver, and the Maldives is one of the world's premier destinations for scuba diving, with its coral reefs, clear warm water, and tremendously diverse marine life. It's sometimes referred to as a "vanishing paradise," because as sea levels rise from the melting of glaciers and icebergs, the Maldives is sinking. Scientists have calculated that if the global climate change trend continues unabated, the Maldives will be completely submerged by around 2045.

I traveled there with Mariela Gomez, who works in the pediatric emergency department at the University of California San Francisco's hospital. Mariela is from Bogotá, Colombia, where she once ran the emergency department in that city's main hospital. She tells stories of how the trauma and carnage was so great that every night would generate a sizeable collection of bodies for the morgue to collect in the morning.

I was also meeting Hamza Alduraidi in the Maldives. He is a classmate from my UCSF nursing PhD program who has become a trusted friend. He lives only a couple hours' flying distance away. After he finished his PhD, Hamza—who had been chosen by his country to study in San Francisco—returned to his native Jordan, where he is now a nursing professor at the University of Jordan.

Before leaving the States, I tried setting up some nursing-related meetings for during my visit. Online, I was able to identify the Maldives Nursing and Midwifery Council, and found a phone number. I called several times, but either no one would answer or the person who did answer would say "yes" to everything I said, and then hang up. So I waited until we arrived in Malé, the capital, and had the hotel staff contact the council for me. Soon we had a meeting scheduled.

Having by now visited a couple of foreign nursing councils, I had come up with a group of questions that I typically ask. They aim at getting a feel for the major issues going on with a council and a country. I want to know about the government agencies that regulate nurses, how many nurses there are, what kinds of salaries they earn, and whether there are nurse practitioners in addition to registered nurses. I ask about foreign nurses—whether they work in the country and how many there are— and about whether the country's own nurses travel abroad to work. Is there a union? Are there male nurses? I like to know about the hospitals: are they private or run by the government?

It was in sweltering tropic heat when Hamza, Mariela, and I walked the two blocks from our hotel to the building that housed the council. We were ushered into the office of Ahlam Ali for our meeting.

In addition to the questions I typically ask, I've also developed a method to these meetings. The important thing is to establish a relationship with the individual I'm meeting with and, by extension, the organization. I've learned over time that it is the key to being able to contact them again with other questions.

I asked Ms. Ali about the council's work and how large an organization it is. The question seemed to confuse her a little. As she explained things, I realized that the "council" was actually one person, and it was *her*.

I learned that most nurses in the Maldives come from other countries, particularly Sri Lanka. Ahlam described the difficulties of regulating nursing in a country in which everyone is spread across more than a thousand islands. Nurses cannot easily come together for meetings or classes.

I asked Ahlam a question that has become routine in my interviews with nursing leaders in other countries: How many male nurses are there in your country? Her answer was four. I pressed a bit: Do you mean 4 percent of nurses in the Maldives are male? No, she said, there are four guys in the entire country working as nurses. And she knows each of them.

After my trip to the Maldives, my next stop was Sri Lanka. It's also an island country in the Indian Ocean, but much larger than the Maldives and much closer to the Indian subcontinent. Many people know the nation by its old name, Ceylon, which it changed in 1972. Independent from British colonial rule only since 1948, Sri Lanka spent 26 years engaged in a bloody civil war that ended in 2009, although sectoral violence is still ongoing.

Again, Mariela and I were only able to make a nursing connection after arriving. Hamza could not join us because of the difficulty for him as a Jordanian to get a visa. This would become an ongoing problem. The hotel staff helped us track down the right people, and we went to the Ministry of Health to meet with the person described as the Chief Nurse in the country's Department of Education, Training & Research. We were told she was on her way and asked to wait for an hour, which we did—in the Ministry's cafeteria, where flies swarmed and the restroom was abysmal. An older man who seemed to work there came over and was chatting. After a few minutes, he asked me for my contact information. He had a 17-year-old daughter who would like to go to the U.S. to study.

"Can you arrange that?"

"No, sorry," I said. "That's not something I can do."

Once the Chief Nurse returned, my meeting started. I introduced myself and told her I was researching nursing regulations in different countries. She nodded and said "yes."

I continued to explain. "Comparing regulatory systems is useful to see how ..." Wait. I noticed she just kept nodding and saying "yes." So I stopped and asked whether I was making any sense.

"Yes," she said, nodding her head again.

I realized there was no polite way to ask my next question. "You don't really speak any English, do you?" But I decided that if she didn't understand what I was saying, then what I was saying was not impolite.

She continued to nod and say "yes."

At that point, I used the usual international signs of smiling to show my gratitude and graciously ended the meeting.

A year later, bombs blasted through some of the hotels and other sights I visited in the capitol city of Colombo on this trip. I can clearly picture the people I had met, and hotel staff, and wonder whether they survived. This has become something of a sad routine, where violence hits in places that I've visited, making it a lot more personal and not just another news headline. The incidents in Sri Lanka were the only ones in countries to which I've made nursing-related visits, but before my career transition, working for the United Nations in East Timor in 1999 (where I registered voters in a small village to vote on independence from Indonesia), or in my personal travels, several places I visited—including Tajikistan, Syria, and elsewhere—and in which I made personal connections with communities were later hit with violence

Two months later, in April 2018, I traveled to Vietnam. Every country faces a unique mix of challenges. The country is very poor, still under Communist control, but is opening up to capitalist methods and has one of the fastest-growing economies in the world. Connecting with a nurse leader in Vietnam would also be challenging.

I sent emails to the Vietnamese Nursing Association that went unanswered. I also contacted Dr. Greg Crow, an RN and nursing professor at the University of San Francisco (USF), who in 2007 established the Vietnam Nurse Project, an academic service partnership between the USF School of Nursing & Health Professions and healthcare workers in Vietnam. Greg had experience working with the nurse leaders and the Vietnam Nurses Association (VNA).

The Vietnam Nurse Project takes American nurses to Vietnam to provide education and training. Each year, a USF delegation visits hospitals and nursing schools in Vietnam and spends a few weeks teaching cutting-edge nursing techniques. As one of the American instructors in the program, though, makes clear, "We aren't trying to turn Vietnamese nurses into American nurses or prepare them to the United States to practice."*

These visiting instructors have found a few key differences between nursing in the two countries. For example, physicians play a key role in running Vietnam's nursing schools, whereas nurses themselves run the nursing profession in the United States. In fact, in the United States, the nursing profession considers it important to avoid even the *appearance* of being under the direction of MDs. Even physician assistants, who can be mistaken by patients as similar to nurse practitioners, are not nurses and do not work in the nursing chain of command. Further, Vietnam has no national nursing law, and legal standards vary dramatically depending on where in the country a nurse is working. Vietnamese nurses have limited scope of independent practice.

Greg warned me that personal contacts were key in Vietnamese society, so I should not expect a response from an organization if they don't know me. He was kind enough to introduce me to Bich Luu Nguyen, who had recently retired from her government job at the Ministry of Health in Hanoi and was working as an advisor to the VNA.

I arrived to meet Ms. Nguyen at the office of the Vietnamese Nursing Association. I'd been given an address that consisted of an entire city block in Hanoi. The taxi dropped me off, but I had to walk around looking for the right building. By the time I found her office, I was soaked with sweat, which was dripping down my face. The assistant took one look at me and asked whether I'd like some water. The water was warm!

Ms. Nguyen described to me her several decades as a nurse in Vietnam. When she began her career, there was no such thing as nursing regulation. This is typical in many countries. There seems to be a natural evolution in which the practice of medicine is regulated from the earliest days. After some time—years or even decades—governments see the value of regulating nurses separately from doctors. While I didn't get the entire picture about the regulation of Vietnamese doctors, it was not until the mid-1990s that the government Health Ministry decided it needed a nurse in the government to act as a representative of nursing. The Ministry simply wanted to know what was going on with nurses. Nguyen had extensive personal contacts in the Ministry, so she was asked to work there as an advisor. From that beginning, she created the office in the Vietnamese government that now regulates nursing. She has since been all over the world in her nursing regulator capacity, and hosts lots of representatives from other countries that visit Vietnam to learn how they might help their own nursing professions back home.

One major difference between Vietnam and other countries that I learned is that nurses in Vietnam earn salaries that are quite a bit better than the average Vietnamese worker. That makes nursing a highly sought-after career, and because of that about 10 percent of nurses in Vietnam are male—a number that is growing. There also seems to be a strong nursing association, which boasts thousands of local chapters. I know of no nursing association in any other developing country that is so vigorous. Whereas in some countries they don't particularly appreciate outsiders chiming in on what nurses ought to do, nursing professionals in Vietnam seem to welcome outside support and advice. Nguyen boasted of the VNA's networking with nurses internationally.

A problem I've encountered on many of my trips abroad to study nursing is that there is often a lack of government transparency, and people were not really open to questions and research. I wanted to know more about nursing regulations in Vietnam. I learned that all the nation's nursing regulations and the nursing association's documents exist only in Vietnamese. That makes sense, given that there are virtually no foreign nurses working here. But it also means that outsiders like me trying to learn from Vietnam are restricted to personal accounts such as that offered by Ms. Nguyen.

Perhaps the most remarkable thing I found with Vietnamese nursing is the importance of the nursing association compared to the government regulators. Whereas nursing *boards* dominate the regulatory landscape in the United States, and nursing associations are relatively weak, the reverse seems to be true in Vietnam. The VNA carries a lot of weight, setting standards of professional conduct, improving the clinical skills of nurses, and simply driving the profession forward. It is as if the government, struggling with limited resources, sees that the nursing profession is self-regulating well and thus has delegated this role to the VNA.

One thing that struck me had to do with the VNP specifically not preparing nurses in Vietnam to work in the United States. What I've observed with nursing around the world is that if a nurse gains enough skills and becomes fluent in English, it can often be very hard to keep her in her home country. The VNP is helping train Vietnamese nurses, but it seems a conscious decision not to train them so well that they might leave Vietnam.

A month after visiting Vietnam, in April 2018, I traveled to Poland and Lithuania. I hoped to learn about nursing regulation in Eastern European countries since the dismantling of the Soviet bloc.

Poland was one of the earlier countries to join the ICN, in 1925. As the organization's fourteenth member, the country's nursing association represented the first Eastern European country to join. Today, it has the strongest economy of all the former Soviet bloc nations. Unfortunately, my best efforts to connect with nursing regulators or professional associations before arriving there had all been in vain. So I resorted to my backup plan: book myself a room in a hotel that caters to businesspeople and ask the staff to help me make nursing contacts. Helping guest with these sorts of business matters is a service some hotels offer routinely. It's not something you can try at just *any* hotel.

In Warsaw, Poland's capital, the hotel's front desk staff made many phone calls both to the nursing council and Poland's nursing association, all without any response. I found the lack of response odd. After the visit, when I mentioned to nurse executives in other European countries my inability to connect with the nurses there, they were surprised. A few

European nurse leaders mentioned to me that Polish nurses play an active role in European nursing. Perhaps it was just back luck and bad timing on my part.

I chose my next destination, Lithuania, because it is a small country that had been under Soviet occupation for decades but was now looking to Western Europe as a model for its government. I wondered how that would that translate into nursing regulations. Another factor in my decision making was logistics and cost. When I am visiting a country, I always consider where else I might easily get to that could help me in my research.

It had been easy to find the Lithuanian Nursing Association online, but my emails elicited no response. So as I had done in Warsaw, I decided to wait until I could get some help from hotel staff in Vilnius, the capital city.

I checked into the Radisson Blu in what is called *Vilniaus senamiestis*, or the Old Town of Vilnius. It's one of Europe's largest surviving medieval towns, a little bigger than three-and-a-half square kilometers in the larger city. Old Town is an architectural marvel of gothic, renaissance, baroque, and neoclassical buildings all intermixed.

Staff at the front desk were very helpful, and soon had me on the phone with the nursing association's Ausra Volodkaite. We spoke in English. She agreed to meet me at my hotel.

It turns out there are two Radisson Blu hotels in Vilnius, and she assumed I was at the one in the financial district, not in Old Town. So after a short delay, she arrived at my location and we sat down to talk.

An experienced nurse, Ausra is helping develop Lithuania's nursing association, which—starting from nothing—has had to create its own programs. That is not as straightforward as one might think. To an American nurse, it may seem obvious what a nursing association is supposed to do, but that's not necessarily the case in other countries. Prior to Lithuania's independence from the Soviet Union, the government controlled just about everything. There was no such thing as an independent association of any type. With independence, Lithuanian society needed to create, from scratch, organizations that were truly independent from the government.

Ausra told me Lithuania had just graduated its first class of nurse practitioners. "How do you train NPs when there are none to begin with," I asked. Her answer was fascinating.

164

At the time of my visit, there were only 15 NPs in the country, all working without a history or tradition from which to draw. Ausra explained that to figure out what NPs should be legally allowed to do, or should do, and how they should relate with RNs and doctors, the nursing school creating the new program looked at NPs in other countries, specifically in Western Europe. Denmark even sent a delegation of nurses to help Lithuania develop its nursing systems.

It was too early to tell what success the NP program has had since the first cohort had only just finished school and entered the workforce.

I thought about what lessons from this experience in Lithuania might inform nursing in other countries. The one that came to mind is that Lithuania demonstrates that a nursing system can be created from almost nothing. You can draw on things that work elsewhere and leave out the things that don't work.

That's a lesson that is probably too late for the United States, however. U.S. nursing boards certainly have a lot of examples from which to draw—after all, every state has 49 other examples in our one country alone—but we no longer have the opportunity to build systems anew. Today, U.S. nursing boards are burdened by history and precedent. When they do attempt changes, the same questions are always raised, automatically: Where did that idea come from? What is the evidence that it works?

U.S. boards are very averse to change. Lithuania showed me that a country could, though, make drastic changes—one hopes they are improvements—to meet societal needs. But Lithuania was starting without the same kind of burden as in the United States.

Money is certainly an issue for Lithuania's nurses. Nurse salaries there are around US$12,000 a year, which is low by European standards. There's also a language issue: it is a prerequisite to speaking Lithuanian to work as a nurse in the country. Lithuanian nurses who speak other languages can easily find work elsewhere, and if that other language is English, they have a ticket to work in a vast number of places. The country struggles to keep good nurses from leaving. With one short plane ride to the west, as so many Lithuanian nurses have done, they can easily double or triple their salaries.

I was lucky to connect with Ausra. She speaks English, but unlike so many of her colleagues, she's chosen to stay in her home country.

My flight back to California from Lithuania included a 14-hour layover in Denmark, and there was no way I was going to let so much time go by without trying to make some more nursing contacts. I searched online for Denmark's nursing council, but it was not easy to identify any one organization that is comparable to a U.S. nursing board. I did, however, find the Danish Patient Safety Authority, so I employed my simple method of emailing anyone whose address I can find and ask for a meeting. If I can't find a name, I'll send an email to the organization's generic email address. Sometimes I'm just hoping whoever gets the email will read my request and send it along to the appropriate office or individual. In this case, I heard back from Majbritt Codam, who agreed to a meeting. Her reassuring title was Head Nurse.

From Ms. Codam's email response, I could already tell Denmark was going to be different. She asked me what was to be discussed and requested that I please inform her if the meeting was to be canceled, so she could plan accordingly. I thought that was a little cold, but also super-organized.

I flew into Copenhagen late at night. The next morning, before heading to my meeting, I packed for the flight home. The hotel called for a taxi. When it arrived, the driver already had my name and destination on a computer tablet mounted on the dashboard so everyone could see who he was there to pick up. Everything here seemed more organized that anywhere else I had ever traveled.

Then I went to the office of the Danish Patient Safety Authority and met Ms. Codam, who I learned was the head of nurse licensing. She had never encountered anyone studying how nurse regulators operate, and was intrigued by my research. That sort of thing always amazes me. In all my visits to U.S. boards, I have never crossed paths with a single person who researches nurse regulators. The same goes for overseas.

I asked Ms. Codam about European nursing rules. I had assumed there is someone at the EU level that sets Europe-wide standards, but I found out that that is not at all the case. As for compliance with those rules, she told me that there is one woman in the Danish government that acts as coordinator for any EU compliance issues.

As it turns out, the Danes have some of the same problem as the Lithuanians. It's hard for nurses from elsewhere to come to Denmark to work, because one needs to speak Danish to be licensed and it is not a common language for foreigners to know. If a Danish nurse speaks another language, she can easily work elsewhere. Because of this,

Denmark struggles to keep good nurses in the country. It's not that working as a nurse in Denmark is bad or that the wages are low (wages are among the best in the world). It's simply that having that second language gives the nurse more options than a Danish nurse that only speaks Danish.

She described for me the process of getting a nursing license in Denmark. Foreign training and diplomas are reviewed, and the quality of an educational program may be investigated. The newly certified nurse is then placed in a probationary role in which she works in a clinical setting while her skills and performance are assessed. Only after several months is she fully licensed to work as a nurse.

One thing that interests me in particular as I study nursing in other countries is what U.S. boards might learn from other nursing regulators. I was thinking about how organized the Danes are in their licensing system, in their regulatory agencies, and everything else I saw on my visit. I don't know how this could be applied to U.S. boards. It's difficult to take one aspect of a system and apply it to another with good results, and so I can't assume anything about Denmark's system could simply be passed along to our U.S. counterparts. Still, an overarching question has continued to linger in my mind: Why are they so organized in the first place and some U.S. boards so disorganized?

There is another important group in Denmark with which nurses are involved: the *Dansk Sygeplejeråd* (DSR), known as the Danish Nurses Organization (DNO) in English. Founded in 1899, the DNO is a voluntary membership organization that counts about 85 percent of the country's practicing nurses—about 77,000—as members. It functions both as a professional association and as a trade union, much like its sister organization in New Zealand.

The DNO has an interesting motto: "We move boundaries—in the organization, profession and society." This leads to activities focused on the internal life and democracy within the DNO itself, as well as on the salaries and working conditions of nurses, as well as on the nursing profession as a whole. "We focus on health political issues, development and research in nursing, and cooperation with other organizations, national and across international borders."[2]

In my limited time in Denmark, I did not have an opportunity to visit the DNO. But it is worth saying a bit more about the organization, especially since it plays an important role through its international collaboration with other nursing groups throughout the world. The DNO hosted the founding congress of the Nordic Nurses' Federation in Copenhagen in 1920, which brought together representatives from the Finnish, Swedish, Norwegian, and Danish associations of nurses, and expanded a few years later to include the Icelandic nurses' association (much later, nurses from the Faroe Islands joined the collaboration).

The Danes were also central to the establishment of several other international nursing groups, including, among others, the European Federation of Nurses Associations, "established in 1971 to represent the nursing profession and its interests" as what would eventually become the European Union was being forged.[3] The DNO also is a leading member of the European Federation of Public Service Unions.

In addition, the DNO engages in what it calls "solidarity work" (*Solidaritetsarbejde*) through its Solidarity Fund that takes a tiny portion of nurse salaries for a pool of money to help nurses who become ill or find themselves in an "economically vulnerable situation," as well as to support efforts in other countries. Most particularly, the DNO collaborates with the nursing organization in Swaziland and other groups to support a health center in the city of Manzini (the country's second-largest city) for healthcare workers and their families. The health center, led by nurses, also reaches out to more rural areas of Swaziland to test health personnel for HIV/AIDS, distribute medications, and examine and treat other diseases. As I mentioned earlier, Swaziland is wracked by HIV/AIDS.[4]

Danish nurses seem to care about nursing and nurses at every level throughout the world, from their professional lives as healthcare providers to their lives as members of society who need access to health services for themselves profession.

I only learned of the role played by the Danes after visiting Denmark—a lesson that I need to do more homework before traveling to a given country. Had I known about the work of the Danish nurses in Swaziland, I would have had more of an impetus to meet with nurses when I was there. My emails to the DNO went unanswered. Here was another learning point for me. In the rarified atmosphere of nursing leadership, even with a high functioning organization like this one, a personal contact is still needed.

Returning home to the United States, it was time to work in earnest on my most elaborate research travel yet: a trip I was planning for January

2019 to study the countries of the Cooperation Council for the Arab States of the Gulf, which aims eventually to be roughly like the European Union, with a common currency, common defense, and so on.* My aim was to see how these countries regulate the nursing profession and how they treat nurses, not only as workers but also as people.

The Persian Gulf countries have a lot of money, and they hire tens of thousands of nurses, mostly from India, Philippines, and Pakistan, attracting them with salaries far in excess of those they could earn in their own countries. Many of these foreign nurses come to the Gulf countries directly from graduation from nursing school; they gain their first non-school experience in these Arab states and often move on to jobs in the United States or Europe. I wondered, therefore, what quality of nursing experience they get working in the Gulf States.

The trip would be essentially the same, I thought, as visiting the U.S. nursing boards, but involving multiple countries. I had asked Hamza, my Jordanian friend from UCSF, to join me. In his work at the University of Jordan, his research has focused on the health status of Palestinians. It's a research area with a personal angle for Hamza, whose mother is Palestinian and father is Jordanian. Mixed parentage of this sort is common in Jordan, which has more refugees as a percentage of its total population than any country in the world—including not only the 1.9 million Palestinians (more than 337,000 of whom live in the country's 10 official refugee camps) but also growing numbers of Syrians who have fled the ongoing war there.

Hamza had jumped at the invitation. Gaining a better understanding of how a government's regulations affect the ability of nurses to do their jobs would help him in his broader research. And so, when we were together in the Maldives, we hatched our plans for the trip over dinner at an Indian restaurant in Malé. We would visit each of the Arab Gulf States to interview anyone who would talk to us—government regulators, hospital administrators, nursing leaders, and nurses.

In advance of that trip, we would go to Geneva, Switzerland—a

---

* Originally called the Gulf Cooperation Council (GCC), a name still widely in use, the council—first established in 1981—serves as a regional economic union and political union for its current members: Bahrain, Kuwait, Oman, Qatar, Saudi Arabia, and the United Arab Emirates (that is, all the Arab states of the Persian Gulf except for Iraq).

major stop on the journey to nursing's decision makers. The city is home to some of the most important global organizations dealing with health, diplomacy, and world power. I wanted to meet with folks at the World Health Organization (WHO), the International Council of Nurses, and the International Labour Organization (ILO). My view is that if you want to understand these organizations, you have to be there in person, see the offices, and meet officials on their home turf. So, I made appointments for Hamza and me to meet in September 2018 with anyone willing to see us at these organizations and headed to Geneva.

In the meanwhile, before meeting me in Geneva, Hamza began networking within the Arab region.

In the run-up to all of us meeting at the beginning of January in the region, Hamza hit the road, beginning to make connections with people we thought could help. In June 2018, he visited the WHO's Middle East office in Cairo, Egypt, where he met Arwa Oweis, a Jordanian nursing professor who is also the WHO's lead person for the region. Her name always came up whenever I made contact with nursing leaders in Geneva or anywhere else in the world. She was the "go-to" person for the Middle East, people would say. We knew that contacts in the region would make all the difference in getting answers to our questions, and thought Arwa would be able to make direct contacts with others on our behalf. But as helpful as she was when it came to giving Hamza lots of pointers about how to organize our study, she could only point to people in the Arab countries she thought we would need to work with.

On more than one occasion later, when we followed up with people Arwa suggested, those same people would tell us we needed to talk to Arwa. It was like a child asking one parent for something, only to be told to talk to the other parent. Government officials and nursing leaders that could not or did not want to answer our questions but also didn't want to be too frank about their inability too discuss these issues found it convenient to deflect us by sending us back to her.

I get it: nurses face hurdles wherever they work. In California, I need to deal with a regulatory system that includes a nursing board that can take my license for any one of a multitude of infractions. Simply being investigated would put a negative mark on my record. Hamza works in Jordan, a country regarded as being among the best in the Arab world in terms of nursing professionalism, with a regulatory body and published rules. Jordanian nurses are well regarded internationally. But even Hamza must contend with a political environment in which his job depends on staying in the good graces of certain powerful individuals.

As I began to get a picture in my mind of what nurses in Arab countries must contend with, it became apparent that protecting "sources" would have to be a top priority. We would not identify the people we contacted except if absolutely necessary, and then in a limited manner. I was not at much risk, because the research trip wouldn't affect my employment in California and I was cautiously optimistic my U.S. passport would get me home without too much of a hassle. Hamza was my main concern. He lives in an Arab country, where his livelihood is at stake. Jordan may be among the more tolerant and liberal of the region's countries, but he is still at risk of political retaliation.

But we persevered in our preparations. Hamza's next visit, in August 2018, was to the ILO's Middle East office in Beirut, Lebanon. Things did not turn out so well. When Hamza met with an official there and described what we would be trying to accomplish, her response was nothing more than "well, good luck with that." That's about as far as the meeting went—but, admittedly, I had been warned.

I had already contacted another ILO official in India that works on the movement of healthcare workers internationally. In our meeting on Skype, she reminded me that the ILO is an organization of member nations, and if the government of an ILO member nation doesn't want people poking around in the country asking questions or making criticisms, it can see to it that a study just doesn't happen.

I wondered how all this might bode for our visit together to Geneva. Any major project is going to have its hiccups, and preparing for that trip was no exception.

Our original plan had been for Hamza to join Mariela and me in Geneva so we could present our ideas for the Gulf States research trip to people we would meet at international organizations and, we hoped, get some support. Our plan was to fly into Paris and then drive to Geneva. It would be cheaper than flying directly to Geneva and also give Hamza his first-ever trip to France. The French consulate in Amman told him 20 days should be plenty of time to apply for what is called a "Schengen Visa," which is a single visa that allows you access to 26 European countries.

Hamza walked into the French consulate, where he learned that the deciders would need 45 days, which had never been mentioned. They would not even accept his application.

Without Hamza, Mariela and I headed to Geneva to connect with the nursing powers that be. First up was the ICN, a federation of national nurse associations from more than 130 countries. It is the world's number-one nursing organization, and one of the oldest—established in 1904 by representatives of nursing associations of the United Kingdom and Northern Ireland, the United States, and Germany. Individual nurses don't join, but the American Nurses Association is a member.

In its first few decades, when the ICN would hold global meetings every four years or so, the organization's growth in country memberships would come from a couple of national nursing associations joining each time. Current member organizations would vote on admitting these new members, which was seen as an important process. As politics would change, or when two world wars broke out, some country organizations would fall away—but they almost always rejoined when things settled down.

These global get-togethers are now held every two years. First there's a conference open to any nurses as individuals, and then an ICN congress at which each member country's nursing association is officially represented.

English-speaking countries dominate the ICN, but that doesn't mean other countries aren't involved. Nurse leaders from non-English-speaking countries simply don't seem to play as active a role because of the communication challenge. The international gatherings are largely in English: one upcoming conference features speakers almost exclusively from Britain, its ex-colonies, and South Africa, although at the biennial conferences there are limited sessions in Spanish and French, with translation offered. Still, it's just easier to participate in the discussions if you speak English—and large numbers of nurses can't be expected to travel long distances to attend a meeting in a foreign language. Nurses from countries where English is not common don't seem to be as attracted to the prospect of attending an ICN conference.

The ICN's office is in a nice building overlooking the lake with Geneva's famous fountain that shoots water a hundred feet into the air. Alessandro Stievano, an Italian professor of nursing who heads up the ICN's research program, was welcoming, gracious, and eager to help— so eager, in fact, that I was floored he tried to accommodate my every request. He even tried to help with my plans to visit the Arab countries to compare how they regulate nursing and treat nurses. I needed contacts in the region and invitations to meet with government officials. Alessandro was happy to do whatever he could—although one major catch is that Saudi Arabia, the most important player in that region, is not a member of the federation.

I find office visits to be quite useful when trying to get to know an organization, and Alessandro gave me a full tour. Often, such a tour reveals an organization's priorities; you see how physical space is organized and how space different people have for their different functions. While the building itself is very nice, ICN's headquarters span two floors of mostly empty offices. There is a staff of 24 people, but I saw only five in the entire place. There were boxes scattered all over and I got the feeling that the ICN was either moving in the middle of a renovation or moving.

I learned from a few ICN staff members, current and former, that compared to other organizations I've visited, ICN struggles to fund its operations. The organization is in a difficult position—it is a non-profit organization that depends on grants and donations for virtually all of its funding. Most of the professional associations that make up the ICN membership are from countries that are not rich; these associations themselves struggle for funds. In turn, the ICN struggles—constantly, I was told—to get them to pay their ICN membership dues. I was told that ICN member associations in the richer countries are continually pushing to be shown how they benefit from paying their dues, putting more pressure on ICN staff. But at the same time, it doesn't seem likely that any of the major countries would leave the ICN, because they feel obliged to be represented in what is viewed as the world's premier nursing organization.

Contrast all these ICN funding issues with nursing boards in the United States, which are government authorities that can force nurses to pay dues in exchange for their licenses. Then there's the Council for Graduates of Foreign Nursing Schools (CGFNS), also in a position to demand money from nurses. Nurses from outside the United States who want to work in this country need to have their foreign professional education and licenses verified. When I visited the Council's Philadelphia headquarters in 2018, the day after attending a meeting of Pennsylvania's nursing board, I was amazed by the spacious, luxurious offices on multiple floors of a building in the heart of the city, adjacent to the

University of Pennsylvania. I cannot recall seeing any other offices as fine as theirs, and thought about that as I visited the ICN's comparatively much sparser headquarters.

As a result of this chronic underfunding, the ICN struggles—as I learned from Alessandro and others—to keep staff, and to keep them in their positions for long periods. Before ever visiting Geneva, I had heard about this high turnover from nursing leaders I had spoken with. And sure enough, not a single member of the ICN staff whose name had been mentioned to me during visits to U.S. nursing boards were still there by the time I arrived in Geneva.

By everyone's account—both ICN staff members and others collaborating with the ICN with whom I've spoken—the work is fascinating and rewarding. In her biography for a speaking engagement at a major ICN conference, one past ICN president mentions that she visited 50 countries during her tenure. But if the pay is so low that ICN staff members cannot pay the bills and support their families, their time on the ICN staff will be short. I saw this in my own work with the United Nations in East Timor in 1999, getting paid about five times less than what would be needed for me to maintain even a modest standard of living when I returned home to California. No matter how important the work may be, recruiting and keeping good people will always be a problem if an organization cannot provide its staff a sufficient salary.

Observing the financial struggle of the ICN, which plays an important international role, reinforced my view that we should support our professional associations and that they, not boards, ought to control the nursing profession. ICN ought to have vastly more funding than it receives. But it doesn't have any of the regulatory control that can be used to force anyone to pay dues.

Our next visit was to the WHO, the specialized agency of the United Nations that focuses on public health around the world. Its large building, which is the center of power in the world of healthcare, stands in sharp contrast to the offices of the ICN. When you visit a place like the WHO, the massive building and the presence of security officers make clear that it is a place of importance. Being late is not an option, and so we arrived with time to find the last parking space in the entire visitor's lot.

European streets and parking spaces are notoriously small. As I nudged my rented Peugeot into the space, a bicyclist yelled, "It's so tight!"

"Yeah, no shit, Sherlock," I thought to myself.

To get into the WHO headquarters, you have to relinquish your passport, which they hold hostage for the duration of your visit. We turned ours over and were met at the security gate by Carey McCarthy, a Chicago native who heads up WHO programs related to nursing and was my host. Unlike at the ICN, we didn't get past the lobby—where we found a table at which to meet.

Carey described what the WHO does in terms of nursing. My main objective for meeting with someone from the WHO was to get on the organization's radar screen. I explained to her my project to visit the Arab countries to study how they regulate nursing. She asked how I funded my project. When I told her I was self-funded, and didn't have to report to anyone else, and had complete control over whatever I might write up in the end, she had a look of envy. It was the same look I'd seen in so many meetings with nursing board members. In the WHO, everything is politicized, and everything the organization publishes is tailored to be inoffensive to everyone.

Thinking about the WHO, I had the same concern as I always have with nursing boards and the nursing profession as a whole. We are dealing with lots of controversial issues. Nurses are stuck in the middle and often suffer when accusations are made or mistakes happen. Yet, the organizations that play important roles, from the state Boards to the ICN and all the way up to the WHO, are political entities that need to placate critics and not offend anyone. The WHO is charged with improving the health of people worldwide. I cannot think of a more demanding mandate. Doing anything that involves bringing people together from all countries, cultures, and languages is a daunting task. The WHO has to do all that even before it can move on to the greater challenge of addressing health.

I was reminded of my visits to the United Nations headquarters and was amazed at how dysfunctional the organization can be. When I was in the Office of the UN High Commissioner for Human Rights a decade ago, the High Commissioner's secretary told me how they were leaving for a certain region the next day. The particular region doesn't matter. From her office, I went down the hall to a top officer reporting to the High Commissioner who was from that same region and asked him about the trip. He looked puzzled.

"She's going there?" he said. "I didn't know!"

This kind of dysfunction isn't something to use as blame, but rather is a testament to how demanding the work is these people are trying to accomplish, and why when I hear people saying we should pull support from these organizations I always disagree. No, I say, the answer is not to take away support. The answer is to support them even more.

Carey reflected all of this. I could tell she was under lots of pressure working at the WHO, and that what's doing could have a positive impact for nurses the world over. But in the end, there was little she could offer to help me in my trip to the Arab countries. WHO operates like an insider's club, where resources and influence are reserved for their own programs.

The final meeting of my Geneva trip was at the headquarters of the International Labour Organization, the UN agency that deals with social protections, international labor standards, and the objective of work opportunities for all. In fact, the ILO predates the United Nations by nearly three decades. In 1919, the ILO was founded "in the wake of a destructive war, to pursue a vision based on the premise that universal, lasting peace can be established only if it is based on social justice."[5] After the UN was established in 1945, the ILO became its first specialized agency.

The ILO has a unique tripartite structure that includes government representatives, employers, and employees. Its mandate it to promote decent work conditions and justice for workers.

Despite being a vast organization of 2,700 employees with offices in 40 countries, the ILO has little direct involvement with nurses. Instead, the organizations tend to look at workers by sector, such as healthcare. Programs that help nurses also protect doctors, psychologists, dentists, and the countless other job titles that fall within health providers, broadly defined. One such program is the Decent Work Across Borders, which seeks to promote training of healthcare workers in the Philippines and India so they can work overseas, earn better salaries, and gain valuable experience, and then share their skills when they return—thus improving the healthcare systems in their home countries.

I wanted to discuss my planned trip to the Arab countries, where I would explore the working conditions of nurses. I had been warned by an ILO official in a country that sends nurses to the Arab countries that my research would not be welcomed by governments there were I to mention working conditions and workers' rights.

We were welcomed at the ILO by Umberto Cattaneo, a statistician who had come from the World Bank and was studying the flows of healthcare workers around the world. He told me that the ILO had more than a thousand staff members just in its headquarters building and does projects worldwide. Yet, most Americans have never even heard of the organization.

As at the WHO, the politics ran heavy. I learned that my study of the labor conditions for nurses was going to be a political minefield.

The trip to Switzerland was not all meetings, though. I spent the weekend in Interlaken to run the Jungfrau Marathon—26.2 miles with an elevation gain of 7,000 feet. It has been 10 years since my last marathon, and I was about 20 pounds heavier. Still jet lagged and suffering a little stomach problem from the yogurt in Paris, I made it to the halfway point. That was it.

My heart sank as I had to drop out, but it gave me pause to think about what it means to face our limits. There I was in the Swiss Alps, competing in a run and feeling sorry for myself for not finishing. How many people in this world would love to have my problems?

While in Switzerland I learned that later that month the Middle East section of the ICN was hosting a conference in Abu Dhabi. My heart leapt. I figured that the only way to answer my questions on a trip to the Gulf States was to pose them directly to government officials, nursing leaders, and nurse themselves, and I knew having the opportunity to do that would require personal contacts. The timing was perfect, and there was no way was I going to miss a conference with nurses from the region we wanted to study. In one room, I figured, I could contact just about anyone that might help us with information or contacts for the upcoming research trip.

I contacted Hamza about coming to the Abu Dhabi conference—we figured the visa issues that scuttled his trip to Geneva wouldn't come up—and booked us rooms at the Hyatt Capital Gate Hotel, which is listed in the *Guinness Book of World Records* as the world's furthest-leaning hotel. Yeah, whatever. More important was that it was the nice hotel attached to the conference, so the key people would be there.

I wasn't sure what to expect of the meeting, and of nurses in the Arab region generally. Nevertheless, the fact that they were holding this conference was an important sign that they take professionalism seriously. I cannot remember any other region in the world holding a similar ICN conference.

The first morning began with the usual ceremonies, which in this case included a reading from the Qur'an. Princess Muna of Jordan spoke; she has taken on nursing as a "cause" and has become a sort of patron saint of the profession. From then on, it was a lot of PowerPoint presentations, which got a little tedious. But during the breaks, things got interesting. My hope was to meet as many nurses as possible, contacts we could call on in the coming months for interviews and information. Hamza and I were not disappointed.

We spent three days rubbing elbows with the chief nurses of a few Arab countries. We met the chief nurse of Saudi Arabia. I figured that would be an important contact from a country tightly controlled when it came to outsiders visiting, but whether these casual meetings would turn into invitations to visit remained to be seen. Both Saudi Arabia and Kuwait require such an invitation to get a visa.

Some of the nurses from Arab countries were dressed in Western-style professional attire and some in local, Arab-style clothing. There was also a large number of fully veiled women at the conference. I had never been in a meeting alongside fully veiled women. I wondered how one participates in professional activities if you can't show your face, but there they were, doing just that.

A Kuwaiti nursing professor who was fully veiled, with only her eyes showing, gave one of the presentations. Kuwait was one of the countries in which we had no contacts, and so after the Kuwaiti's presentation was over, I approached the front of the room to talk with her. There was a bunch of women around her, all veiled in the same black fabric, and in an instant she blended into the crowd. I could not figure out which one of the women was her, and it seemed inappropriate to just call out her name.

In the hallway a short while later, I was talking to a nursing executive I knew and told her of my predicament. She looked around, spotted the Kuwaiti in the crowd, and called her over. I introduced myself and told her of our plans to visit Kuwait. She said that would be great, and grabbed a nursing professor friend of hers, also veiled, who gave me her card. Funny how the one that just gave a presentation to a room full of nursing professionals did not feel she could be a contact herself. It was the first time ever I had spoken to veiled women.

The conference was the most ethnically mixed of any meeting I've attended. In addition to representatives of the Arab states, there were lots of Filipinos and Indians, since they make up the bulk of the region's nursing labor force. Of Westerners present, the British were predominant.

The conference proceedings revealed that nurses are not the submissive order takers that are the stereotype of some regions. That pleased me. The presentations and projects were as ambitious and professional as anywhere else in the world.

Still, by the end of the conference, I had noticed a few things. One was that nurses in the Middle East avoid controversy, just as they do everywhere else in the world I have visited. There were no debates and no presentations on any topics that would invite opposing views. Second, while the proceedings revealed that nurses are taking on far more than they can handle, the speakers kept encouraging us to continue taking on even more work. Annette Kennedy, the ICN's head, gave the first presentation. She spoke of global problems and how nurses can help solve them. War, poverty, global warming—the list went on and on.

To my mind, nurses are already overworked and overextended, yet here were nurse leaders telling us to add all these things to our to-do list. That night, in my hotel room, I was flipping through the latest edition of *American Nurse Today*. There was an article on loneliness and how nurses need to assess patients for loneliness. Jeez, this never ends!

I made a lot of contacts in Abu Dhabi, and when I returned home to California I began sending emails and making phone calls. First up was the chief nurse of Saudi Arabia, who had been quite pleasant when I met him at the conference and expressed interest in our project. We needed a visa to visit Saudi Arabia, and that required an invitation. I thought he would be the perfect person to invite us. But I received no response.

I went online and researched Saudi nursing academics and government administrators. I found a Saudi government official who was responsible for training and hiring healthcare professionals. On his LinkedIn account, he even mentioned all the thousands of foreign healthcare workers he brought to his country. So I contacted him about an invitation and a visa.

"Sorry," he told me, "I am not able to do that."

I was stunned. According to his résumé, it seemed to me that that was exactly what his job entails.

Hamza and I were also still having trouble fulfilling another need we had identified for our research trip. We wanted to find a female Arab nurse to accompany us. It wasn't lost on us how this quest might appear. Nursing is already a predominantly female profession, and here were two guys trying to understand what is going on in a part of the world where the sexes—not just in nursing—are more divided than just about anywhere else. Still, though, we had put the word out at the conference to everyone, and we thought we would find someone. But while a few expressed interest, we ultimately had no luck. We began to think we could settle for a female nurse from somewhere else but who could speak Arabic.

After the conference, not having found anyone, we turned to our professional networks and ended up inviting an Arab woman with a nursing PhD from a top university and a long list of awards for her nursing research. She expressed interest but wanted to know more. So I arranged a meeting for the three of us on Skype. Hamza and I were on video, but she phoned in. We couldn't see her face. I wondered: Was this a matter of not having video capabilities, or did she not want us to see her?

In my email, I had mentioned the risks associated with the project, and now I explained to her that any study of government activity in the Arab region, no matter how innocuous, needed to be done with care. Hamza stated that as long as our intentions were noble and our research methods were sound, all would be fine.

Not so, the woman declared. She described a recent research proposal she had submitted to her own university. The university had paid a lot of money for an accreditation, and she wanted to see whether being accredited had improved anything. In other words, she was asking whether her school got anything for its investment of time and money. The dean called her, demanding she withdraw the proposal. The leadership did not want to entertain a research proposal that could reflect negatively on the school. This, she said, was an example of how our project would involve political dangers even in academia or nursing— that is, beyond the more obvious ones with governments.

A couple of weeks later, she declined to join us. So it was time for Plan B: find a female nurse regardless of Arabic language skills.

A few weeks after the Abu Dhabi conference, in early October 2018,

Mariela and I made a trip to the Republic of Georgia, where we met with a remarkable nurse named Ia Gelenidze who was working in a country with virtually no nursing regulations. As of this writing, Georgian nurses are not licensed; the government has enacted no nursing legislation; and hospitals have to figure things out on their own in terms of what nurses should do. Ia leads an organization, Future Nurses, that advises the government and hospitals on how to manage nurses and the nursing process. She looks to other countries for examples, but in Georgia she has to make these professional standards work in a society where nurses do not have a license at stake. It was great that Ia agreed to join us on our trip to the Arab states.

Also joining us was Mariela, who has traveled to about a quarter of the world's countries. We've often been together in meetings with nursing leaders in far-flung places. She's been to North Korea as part of a delegation of people from more than forty countries. In a CNN International broadcast, a North Korean authority being interviewed about the visit said, "We even have someone from Colombia!"

On Mariela's trips, being a woman often gains her access to places and people I could not. In Afghanistan, for instance, she was able to see what happens in rooms where no men are allowed.

So, it was set: our "delegation" to the Gulf States would be Hamza, Ia, Mariela, and me.

Mariela and I had already visited the ICN, WHO, and ILO in Geneva, but it was important for Hamza and Ia as well to make themselves known to the powers that be there. I asked them to visit in December, just before the Arab trip.

Again, Hamza had visa problems—just as when we tried to meet in France. This time the problems were with Switzerland directly. Then, because he had requested a tourist visa, the French government had been under no obligation to give him any reason for saying no. This time, he had a letter of invitation from the ICN, prepaid round-trip tickets, and hotel reservations. But still he was denied. The Swiss informed him in a letter that the denial was because he "failed to show adequate financial means."

I was amazed by this turn of events. I could fly into Europe with no visa and no restrictions, but here was a nurse, a professor at his nation's top university with a PhD from a prestigious American university, who wanted to come to Europe because he was volunteering his time on a research project intended to benefit all of our healthcare knowledge, and he faced insurmountable hurdles. The Swiss ultimately denied him that opportunity.

To appeal that decision, Hamza would need to hire a specialist immigration lawyer in Switzerland and then pay additional fees for a reapplication. He reckoned all that would cost almost a year's worth of his salary. This, he explained to me, is the plight of Arab men under the age of 30. No matter how law abiding they are, governments around the world routinely treat them as if they pose a security risk, until proven otherwise.

Ia went to Geneva, without visa problems, and met with the ICN's top people. Georgia is not an ICN member state, so my theory was that she would be well received: the ICN is always interested in bringing in new members. Ia has been ambitiously trying to build nursing professionalism in her country, and they offered to help her however possible.

As the time for our Gulf States trip got closer, we tried repeatedly to contact government leaders in those countries, as well as nursing academics, and, quite frankly, anyone that would talk to us. Not a single person in Saudi Arabia or Kuwait would agree to a meeting. In the meanwhile, something happened that made international news and raised big questions for us. In October 2018, Jamal Khashoggi, a Saudi dissident and journalist for the *Washington Post*, was murdered at the Saudi consulate in Istanbul, Turkey. Soon, it was revealed that the murder was likely premeditated and carried out by agents under the direct order of Saudi Crown Prince Mohammed bin Salman. The international recriminations that followed put a chill on our planned trip scheduled to begin only a few months later.

The Khashoggi murder, though, was not the only concerning event. The previous May, a British student named Matthew Hedges, who had traveled to Dubai to conduct research on defense policies as part of his PhD program, had been arrested by United Arab Emirates authorities after an Emirati man reported that he had been asking "sensitive" questions and claimed he was trying to obtain classified information. After languishing in jail for six months, he was dragged into a courtroom for a five-minute hearing with no lawyer present and sentenced to life imprisonment for espionage on behalf of the British.

What would happen to us for asking "sensitive" questions, Hamza and I wondered as the Hedges story spread worldwide.

While Hedges was pardoned a week later after the British government's repeated interventions on his behalf finally bore fruit, and he returned to the United Kingdom, the chill we felt was very real. But we persisted with our planning. I found the contact information for the Bahrain Nursing Association on the ICN website and sent an email. I received a cryptic email reply that said the association was shut down and that I should check it out on the Internet. When I did that, I learned that the association president Ms. Rula al-Saffar, had been arrested back in April 2011 when security forces rounded up some 20 doctors, nurses, and paramedics for providing treatment for demonstrators who had been involved in the Arab Spring protests. She later told of how she had been tortured over her four-month detention—shocked with stun guns, beaten, and threatened with rape.

I took note of the fact that Ms. al-Saffar was awarded the U.S. State Department Women of Courage Award. Hamza and I didn't have anything like that in our résumés. What might be our fate in Bahrain for asking questions about nursing?

In the meanwhile, I received an email from an official in Oman in response to my inquiry about visiting that country. He warned me that any study of government regulation was extremely sensitive, and we would need official permission from every country of the Gulf council. I wrote back and asked who I needed to contact about obtaining such permission. Not surprisingly, he never responded.

By December 2018, as the trip approached, we had all come to realize that our study topic had solidified around something rather different than government regulations and their effects on nursing. Instead, it would be a study of how nurses work in a region where regulations are treated like state secrets. And it became clear that telling Hamza and Ia that when they applied for their visas they should make them *tourist* visas—don't mention any research or meetings, I had said— had been good advice.

On New Year's Eve, Mariela and I boarded a plane from San Francisco to Dubai, where we met with Hamza and Ia for what would prove to be a short but informative trip. We had only three meetings set up before arriving in the region: two in the United Arab Emirates and one in Bahrain. They were all with non-Arab individuals, and only one of them was connected to the government.

We had chosen to start in Dubai because the city is the social, economic, and transport hub of the Gulf region. It was no accident: the UAE had built the largest international airport in the world and created a business environment that would be open and tolerant to all precisely for that purpose. But whereas most people probably think of Dubai's glitzy skyscrapers and its decadent resorts, I see Dubai as a place where the world meets—including nursing. And so, if the UAE is a country that wants to cater to the global community, the question of how its nurses are treated is an important one to ask. After all, if there are not clear and well-recognized rules to which everyone needs to adhere, there cannot be a *profession*.

Our first scheduled meeting in the UAE was with two nurse managers in a hospital known for its world-class standards and considered a pioneer in its field. I had met these two nurses at the Abu Dhabi conference a few months earlier. We drove out of Dubai and across the desert to another city where they work. We could see camels on both sides of the freeway. For Ia, who had not traveled much, it was the first time seeing a camel in real life.

We arrived in the hospital and met our contacts in the café for what turned out to be an eye-opening introduction to the region and what nurses working in the UAE face. Both of the nurses are expatriates from Europe, working in the UAE for a short period with no expectation of settling down. Their visas are work visas—as is the case for all the Gulf countries when it comes to expatriate nurses. Further, the Gulf States forbid foreigners from retiring in these countries no matter how long they may have worked or participated in the community.

The country is wealthy enough to recruit nurses from just about anywhere in the world, and for nurses from many parts of the world the pay in the UAE is substantially better than anything that could ever be expected at home. The exact wages depend on some multiplier of those in the nurse's country of origin, or some other formula. Nurses from Philippines, India, or Pakistan, for instance, are paid the equivalent of about US$40 thousand per year in the UAE. An American or European nurse earns 50 percent more than that. If you're a citizen of the UAE, you earn another 50 percent or so more on top of that. These wages do not depend on your skills or experience, just your nationality.

The nurses we met with at the hospital described government regulation in the UAE as essentially non-existent in that whatever is written in any documents is not usually how things play out in real life. It was clear that a well-paid nursing job does not translate into professionalism, by which I mean the ability to advocate for yourself, the patient, or the nursing profession. Nor is there any job security. Nurses were here to work, and work diligently, without complaint. Hospitals hire and fire at will. This confirmed a story I had heard about a nurse working in an executive position in a UAE hospital who, from time to time, would be given a list of staff members that would need to leave the country within 24 hours. No reason was given, and no questions were asked.

A Filipina nurse working in a rural area makes as little as US$100 a month in her home country, but many times that in the UAE. Why would she risk everything to speak up? I was beginning to understand why getting any nurses to agree to talk to us had been so difficult. The fact that these two were doing so now was admirable.

As our meeting ended, I had a question that had nothing to do with nursing. Mariela and I had seen plenty of camels in our travels, and Hamza was from Jordan, but Ia seeing camels on our drive had created a desire to see them up close. Where, I asked, might we do that? They suggested we go to Ikea.

The Swedish furniture store has camels, I wondered aloud? No. It turned out that the camel market was located just behind the Ikea. We found scores of camels there, and the camel tenders were more than eager to let us get up close. Ia got to meet camels.

The next morning we visited the one government official—also an expatriate—that had agreed to meet. I was surprised she would talk to us.

We arrived at the government office building, which was quite luxurious, and were soon ushered into her office. She had worked in the UAE for more than ten years and seemed comfortable in her position. I took the fact that a woman was in her position to be an encouraging sign. I struggled to figure out exactly what it was she did, because job titles and actual authority to make decisions seem quite fluid in the region. She manages the licensure and oversight of nurses in that Emirate, but her day-to-day duties seemed to involve a lot more politics than mere administration.

She told us a little more about the differential treatment of nurses depending on whether they are from rich countries, poor countries, or are Emirati citizens. I was surprised by her candor.

Nursing is considered a lowly position in the UAE, and so it is a struggle to find citizens that want to be nurses. Citizens don't even have to take the exam required of all others to get a UAE nursing license; in fact, they are *forbidden* from taking the exam! All they have to do is request a nursing job, and it's theirs for the asking. And then none of the rules that apply to other nurses apply to these citizen nurses. That is why, she explained, there are lots of nursing positions with vague titles that do not involve patient contact. These are for citizens that don't want to care for patients or lack clinical skills.

"But are nurses and their hospitals held to world-class standards in Dubai?" I asked.

Yes, she said. There are more than 4,000 healthcare-providing institutions (hospitals, clinics, or others), and the government inspects them on a regular basis—including surprise inspections. That was encouraging. But what about the regulations? I always look at enforcement to see whether the rules on the books match what is being enforced; that has always been my concern with nursing in the United States.

She was quite frank. There are new rules that centralize the authority of nursing from the individual emirates to the national government.* However, the local authorities often pay no attention to the national rules. Nurse disciplinary actions are typically initiated by hospitals when a nurse makes a mistake, and the process is not open to public scrutiny.

What I was seeing, as I sit in her luxurious office, was a system with the appearance of transparency and rules but a reality that is from that. I remembered our meeting the prior day, where we learned that a nurse could be fired from her job and removed from her country with no questions asked. But I didn't push our confidante that day on any of that; our trip was just beginning, and I didn't want to put her or my fellow researchers at risk. So I stuck to my usual approach with contacts: asking questions calibrated to get as much information as possible without putting them in awkward or dangerous positions. Instead, I wondered whether she might be able to tell us what had happened in Bahrain, where the Nursing Association had reportedly been shut down and the head

---

* The United Arab Emirates is a federation of seven emirates, each governed by a separate ruler. These rulers comprise the Federal Supreme Council, one member of which serves as president of the UAE.

nurse arrested.

She shook her head and said, "Yes, that's a sad situation." Nothing further was offered.

After those two meetings, Hamza had to return home. Getting the visa for the UAE had been easy, but he didn't succeed with the other countries on our itinerary. Applying for a tourist visa wasn't an option; he needed a letter of invitation. Ia, Mariela and I could simply enter Oman or Bahrain as tourists. Seeing one of the region's most talented nursing scholars being turned away because of his passport was becoming tiresome.

We like to think we are judged for our knowledge, our talents, and our accomplishments. But when it comes to traveling and working internationally, we are mostly judged—at least by governments—by the passports we carry. Mariela is a naturalized U.S. citizen. If Mariela, born in Colombia, had been carrying a Colombian passport, there is little chance she would have been with us on the trip. The visa burdens would have been comparable to those Hamza confronted.

We said goodbye to Hamza and rented a car, reassured by the rental agency that we could drive into Oman. So we headed for the border, a few hours drive, where a customs official told us a rental car could not be taken out of the UAE.

"We were told that that wouldn't be a problem," I protested. But he said the rules had changed—and pointed us to the customs office. We parked and walked in.

I was having visions of having to drive back to Dubai, turn in the car, and book a flight for the three of us to Muscat, Oman's capital. But the customs official told me to go to the other border crossing, an hour's drive away, where they wouldn't care the car was a rental. We took his advice.

I couldn't help but note that we were there to study government regulation of nursing, but we were also getting an eye-opener about how the government runs its other operations. In one short time, we had one government official say a rule had changed—apparently for only one crossing—and another tell us how to get around the rule.

At the other crossing, we entered Oman without a problem.

Oman is quite different from the UAE, and it holds a special place in my heart since my first visit there a decade ago. It's quiet and serene, with almost none of the development and glitz of its neighbors. Omanis that you meet on the streets are friendly and approachable.

We were in Oman despite getting the email warning that any research would need government permission. So our plan was to ask only for information that was publicly available. Since we had no contacts and no appointments, we did the next best thing. We looked on the map for a university, hoping we might meet someone who could help.

The one university we found seemed quiet when we arrived, as if classes were not in session. That's good, I thought, because in my experience there will be some faculty around but they won't be distracted by their teaching responsibilities. We saw signs for the health sciences part of the campus, and then a sign for the nursing school. That was easy.

We walked into the quiet building and asked the first person we met where we could find the dean's office. Then we walked into the dean's office. Staff members sitting at their desks looked at us with surprise.

"I'd like to meet the dean," I said. We were told she wasn't there, but one lady on the staff walked us down the hall to the office of a faculty member who was around. We walked into her office.

She, too, was surprised. She apologized for having forgotten about our appointment. I assured her that there was no missed appointment and no planned meeting, and that we really had just showed up at her office. Okay.

We ended up having a great meeting. She was gracious and helpful, answering all our questions as best she could. Like the nurses and official we had met in the UAE, she was an expatriate, not from Oman. She confirmed that government regulations are not typically published, and that Oman has no nursing legislation.

In Oman, we learned, nursing is considered a good career—quite a difference with the UAE. That means there is a large number of Omanis applying for admission to the nursing school. I asked about male nurses—in the UAE, it is rare for a male to be among the few Emiratis that enter the nursing profession—but in Oman things are quite different. The school has to limit the number of males admitted, because so many apply that if there was no limit the number of male nursing students would be much greater than women. The professor told us that each incoming class is 30 percent male and 70 percent female.

When I pressed for an explanation of the percentages, and wondered why it wasn't 50–50, she said she didn't know where the percentages came from.

At one point, she found in her piles of papers a booklet on Oman's nursing code of conduct and said we could keep it. I read it later: it was largely generic, based on ICN and other Western codes. It said nurses should work hard and be held accountable for their actions—essentially what it says in every country's code of conduct. But I wondered whether the government authorities or nursing leaders are similarly held accountable for their actions? It's the same concern I always have with nursing regulators, whether they're in the United States, the Arab world, or anywhere else. Nurses are being held accountable for all our actions, and the nursing profession is energetically pushing for more and more accountability, while our managers, leaders, and government regulators are not being subjected to anything close to the same sort of scrutiny. As for Oman, the country did not publish its nursing regulations, would not allow us to ask openly about the situation, but did publish a booklet calling for nurses to adhere to this stringent code of conduct.

I had one last question before we left this nursing professor. I asked her if she could tell me anything about the situation in Bahrain. Just as the nurse official in Dubai had done, she shook her head and said it was a tragic situation. Nothing further was said.

Oman had to be Ia's last part of the trip, given her hectic work schedule. That last night, we had dinner at a restaurant in Muscat's old city, on the port. Seated at the other tables were some locals and lots of tourists. I enjoy traveling as a tourist, but it's important to me that my visits matter for something more than a few pictures in the album. My research has allowed me to experience things in the countries I've visited that tourists would not see and probably care little about, if at all. Oman is a beautiful country with friendly people, but like other countries, I found a dark side in the way nurses are treated.

The next morning, Ia flew home. Even if her Georgian passport gave her more access than Hamza's Jordanian passport, there were still problems. She could not get a multiple entry visa for the UAE. So instead of joining Mariela and me for the drive back to Dubai, I had to book her a flight from Muscat with a layover in Dubai and home to Tbilisi. I thought about this: We were four nurse researchers on a short trip to visit these countries, and we always had the option simply to go home and return to our regular jobs. Yet we were having major problems with visas and access. Imagine how much harder it must be for a nurse from a poor country trying to get to one of these Arab countries to earn a living. She doesn't have a U.S. passport to gain easy access to most countries of the world, and she needs that job to support a family.

It was left to Mariela and me to go to Bahrain. It was the most concerning country of the visit. Before embarking on the trip, I had sent emails to two universities that offered nursing programs. In my message to the University of Bahrain, I requested a visit, and a professor wrote back asking me the purpose of my trip. I responded with an explanation of our research, and I heard nothing back.

The other contact was with the Royal College of Surgeons in Ireland (RCSI), which has a campus in Bahrain—which may seem odd. But it turns out, according to the RCSI website, that the Irish university has a "long-standing history of educating Bahraini students," and so was invited to set up it own campus in the country. What was opened in 2004 with a cohort of 28 medical students is, as of this writing, "home to a student body of more than 1,300" in schools of medicine, nursing and midwifery, and postgraduate studies and research.[6] I sent an email, and one of the nursing professors soon responded, welcoming us to visit the campus. Faculty from that school had been at the Abu Dhabi conference—a good example of how international nursing conferences play an important role in connecting the nursing community.

It is a short 90-minute flight from Dubai to the tiny Kingdom of Bahrain, which is a small archipelago centered around Bahrain Island. We passed the nursing school at the university—a prominent new building next to the freeway—on our taxi ride from the airport into the center of Manama, the capital.

The next morning, we went to our appointment with the nursing professor. We arrived at the edge of the campus, where guards at a security gate asked us for our names. They looked at a list in their shed, and nodded approval. Once in the building, the nursing professor—another expatriate—met us and led us to her office.

The professor explained that the majority of Bahrain's population is Shiite Muslim, but that the ruling class is Sunni. Conflict between the two is a regular feature of Bahraini life. I learned later that the government has been working for a long time to try to tip the demographic balance of the country in favor of the Sunni minority, stripping Shiites of their citizenship and recruiting foreign-born Sunnis for the Bahraini security forces and giving them citizenship. Security personnel sometimes occupy Shiite villages, restrict Shiite movements, and destroy Shiite property.

I asked about the closing of the nursing association and the fate of its executive director, but the professor had no specific information. She did say that since the time of the Arab Spring demonstrations in 2011, Shiite nursing students have been able to graduate from the school but couldn't get jobs. Some hospitals, including the one right across the street from the university, would hire only Sunnis.

I also asked about nursing regulations. The UAE publishes rules that aren't followed. Oman treats the topic like a state secret. Bahrain, she said, has no published nursing rules. I got the impression that nurses in Bahrain, even more so than nurses in those two other countries, would not feel comfortable making any waves. But to find out, I would need to ask some nurses directly—and I didn't want to push my luck.

As Mariela and I left Bahrain for the return flight to California, I felt that many of my questions had been answered. The lack of rules and regulations tells me a lot. The fact that Saudi Arabia and Kuwait would not let us in speaks volumes. This is a region where nurses are valued, but as a commodity, not as people. They can be disposed of at will.

I find myself wondering how the experience nurses gain working in the Gulf States carries into their jobs in the West. Do they advocate for themselves or for their patients once they're working in American hospitals? Do they feel safe reporting medication errors? I haven't seen any studies to answer these questions.

I do not mean to pick on the Gulf States region as an example of bad nursing regulation. No one involved with New York State's nursing board would talk with me. Staff at the NCSBN hung up on the phone on me when I tried to ask them questions. Clearly, lack of transparency is an issue everywhere, to varying degrees. What does concern me is that nursing community isn't raising more of a concern.

At the September 2018 ICN conference in the UAE's capital city of Abu Dhabi, the topic of nursing regulation had hardly been mentioned. Speakers talked endlessly about how wonderful are and how much everyone loves nurses. Yes, because nurses work to make their patients happy. But simply making that declaration doesn't provide the nurse with respect and job security.

I remembered that one speaker at the ICN conference, a British nursing professor, had specifically thanked the UAE's royal families for their support of nursing. How bizarre and condescending. The support we need, which they don't give in the UAE, is in the form of government regulations that provide us with the rules we need to do our jobs successfully, and enforcement of those rules in a fair and impartial manner.

The 2021 ICN conference is slated for Abu Dhabi again. In other words, a region that provides almost no legal protections for nurses is going to host the meeting of the global nursing community. I hope that by then more of us will be raising our voices.

Chapter 7 References

* Hill and Crow, "Vietnam Nurse Project."
2 Danish Nurses Organization, "Welcome to DNO."
3 European Federation of Nurses Associations, "History."
4 Danish Nursing Organization, "Solidaritetsarbejde.
5 International Labour Organization, "About the ILO."
6 Royal College of Surgeons in Ireland, "About RCSI Bahrain."

8

Moving Forward

Megan, while in a nursing school program, did her clinical rotations in the community hospital's ED alongside Bana, the highly experienced and effective senior nurse. Bana had come from another ED, where things had not worked out so well. As a registry nurse, she had been vulnerable to accusations from anyone that did not like her for any reason. Sherry, the senior nurse who served as her mentor at her previous job, knew Bana was a good nurse with lots of potential, but had fallen afoul of other senior nurses over personality conflicts. But Bana had also watched Sherry's powerlessness when she had to face management over written reports of medication errors that, because they didn't involve patient safety, Sherry had seen countless times go unreported.

Bana is determined to make a change in her new position. She begins attending the department meetings and takes an active role in the union. Hospital management respects her for maintaining an ongoing dialogue so there will be no surprises when problems occur. There are also fewer threats of litigation because both sides, nurses and management, know their ability to resolve disputes will be considered as good-faith efforts if anything ever does end up in court. But no nurse working alone can effect the kind of *fundamental* change needed to make all the nurses in a hospital work with nursing management productively and sustainably.

The *Just Culture* model is floating around the hospital. From time to time, it is in management presentations, only to disappear until the next quality improvement drive or Joint Commission inspection. Bana lobbies her managers, other nurses, and hospital staff to make *Just Culture* an explicit policy, posted on the hospital's website, with a clear statement that no one will be punished for an error without the protections of due process.

Meanwhile, Megan is offered a permanent job in that same ED after completing her program, and decides to stay. Her nursing experience has been limited to the clinicals from nursing school, when senior nurses like Bana (who got credit for her work with her) serve as mentors. Mentors have lighter patient loads, and their performance evaluations explicitly mention the additional role as part of their job duties. Every nurse in the hospital is allowed and encouraged to work at her or his full scope of practice, performing all the skills for which they have knowledge and ability. There is even a program for expanding the range of activities so RNs can fill gaps and meet patient needs. Megan and Bana have also been reaching outside of their hospital, taking an active role in the nursing association. This is where they can meet nurses from other facilities to learn best practices and lobby regulators on issues that affect the nursing profession.

Creating a just culture, putting an end to bullying, promoting a strong labor union, mentoring new nurses, and working at the full nursing scope of practice are ways nurses can fix the problems plaguing us. These might seem like easy fixes, but for Bana and the other nurses already working hard, stressed, and struggling to keep their jobs, these changes take a lot of effort and come with a lot of risk.

For Bana and Megan, the biggest challenge is still in the works. Responding to errors, whether they involve medications or any other matter of patient safety, can be a political landmine. Even the *Just Culture* models used in most hospitals fail to make a clear and public statement that the vast majority of errors do not affect patient safety. But even if safety is affected, the errors are part of a system run by humans, and humans make mistakes. While the other hospitals were sticking to their traditional stance that all errors are documented and vigorously investigated, Bana's hospital would appear to be reckless if it said it would not look into every reported error.

This is where the union comes into play, as a strong partner for Bana and Megan as they advocate for patient safety. If the hospital wants to save money by discharging patients too early, the union helps protect them from retaliation for advocating longer stays. If Megan makes an honest mistake and is worried about losing her job if she files a report, the union helps her know that it won't be so easy for management to fire her.

Add to this story the nursing manager, Cynthia, as well as the hospital executives, the ranks of which rarely include nurses. Cynthia could also be blamed for the decisions she makes, and she also needs protection from bullying, negative politics, and false accusations.

The hospital at which Cynthia, Bana, and Megan work has adopted a worker-management arrangement much like those at Kaiser Permanente and the Veterans Administration. Working together in a partnership like that encourages long-term thinking, not just meeting short-term interests. For instance, it helps everyone see that if nurses push for wage increases that are unsustainable, it will only hurt them in the long run. It helps someone in a management position like Cynthia's that if she wants to employ more registry nurses, it could be seen by regular staff as undermining them, and she may find the flow of ideas and support enjoyed in the partnership evaporates. Under the old system, Cynthia did not appreciate how much of her information came from the nurses giving honest and frank opinions and facts, things that do not normally show up in official documentation.

The story of Megan, Bana, and Cynthia—my only fictional one—suggests a future in which the nursing profession has made adjustments like those discussed in the preceding chapters.

Nursing's Decision Point

The nursing profession has grown and evolved from its beginnings when nurses filled a relatively unskilled role to today, when they are full-scale healthcare *professionals*. I feel we are in a pivotal moment in our evolution at which we now have responsibility for patient care that would have once been unthinkable. In that context, rather than simply carrying out doctors; orders, we need to take control of our patients' program and understand the big picture of their healthcare needs. This means even countering the actions of a doctor if necessary.

What is now missing from this picture is the authority to fulfill our roles. We need to feel assured that our jobs and safety will not be at risk if we take necessary actions that may conflict with other clinicians and/or the hospital administration. Having the responsibility for overall patient care means we should also have the authority to make decisions required to carry out whatever actions may be necessary.

This is where I am concerned about our future. There are some trends that are hurting us now and will continue to undermine us as individual nurses and as a profession.

One is that healthcare-related litigation is increasing. This is not targeted at nursing *per se*; doctors and hospitals also must deal with this. Another is regulation: the government is becoming increasingly specific about what constitutes being a "nurse" and what we are and are not allowed to do. As our job requirements increase, the leeway needed to carry out the tasks is decreasing.

In addition, nurses face a loss of privacy. Our work and personal lives are becoming blurred. Nurses are being disciplined and fired for actions that have nothing to do with their work performance.

Corporate control of hospitals is increasing, and those corporations look to save money—which often includes finding new ways to control staff. Outsourcing is an example: Bana had to work as registry nurses in the hopes of one day getting a secure position.

One of the greatest threats to the nursing profession has been the ongoing attack on labor unions in general. Vast swaths of the United States are so-called "right-to-work" states that outlaw the closed shop— that is, a place of employment that is unionized and everyone must be a member of the union. But the closed shop is what gives the union its power to avoid management's "divide-and-conquer" strategies to break unions. In other places, unionization is made particularly difficult because of the lack of laws and practices that protects workers engaged in membership drives. It's why so many nurses are unorganized, and healthcare-related unions are most likely to be found in Veterans Administration hospitals.

Even in states with strong nurse unions, such as California and Massachusetts, there is a constant battle. Take the University of California–San Francisco Medical Center, a major hospital with a unionized staff. The hospital has received multiple donations of hundreds of millions of dollars, yet it tries to deny benefits and job security to staff at the lowest levels. In other words, a hospital with world-class medical talent often treats everyone but doctors like faceless laborers who can be easily done away with.

When hospitals take positive actions like the labor-management agreement at the hospital where Cynthia, Bana, and Megan work, they often do so in response to a unionization threat. Cynthia, as nursing manager, is well aware that the unions are trying to get into her hospital, and part of her job is to help keep them out. That's why she meets with the nurses and tells them of about what a good working relationship they have and how that would be jeopardized if they voted in a union representing them. Take away the threat of unionization, and I wonder how long that goodwill would last.

Again on Challenges and Solutions

When I was a new nurse at the ED, there were lots of highly qualified nurses working hard but in endless conflict. Even managers were struggling to cope, and most of the nurses were not collaborating as professionals, but functioning in cliques and what nurses often refer to as "mafias." It was like the case I saw come before Nevada's nursing board, in which an LPN's career was under attack by other nurses whose bullying was aided and promoted by the board itself. Meanwhile, the leaders of nursing schools and hospitals were somehow immune to personal responsibility. That nurse in Nevada didn't have the protection of a union, which gives nurses a needed personal advocate so we can perform our jobs with some degree of security.

Job security, though, will only get a nurse so far. The issue of caring keeps coming up: nursing plays a special role in our society, and it is important for us to provide that human touch that turns cold and sterile hospitals into a place of healing. Nurses enjoy the public's trust, but it has prevented us from fulfilling our role as knowledge professionals. We need to combine the caring role with that of a healthcare professional.

So much of how we think about caring is ill founded and misleading. Nurses are already overworked and stressed out, so personalizing our patients' pain is not an answer to what caring should mean. We can do our jobs well without feeling guilty for not having shared tears with our patients. Karen in chapter 2 showed how easy it is to compartmentalize feelings: she felt sympathy for a dying child, but not so much for a manipulative rich male patient. Compartmentalizing our feelings can be a good thing. It helps us with caring, but without letting the stress destroy us.

Then there's "smarts"— all that nurses need to know and demonstrate, particularly when working in a high-stakes environment such as a hospital. Todd (from chapter 3) was a volunteer in the ED, where his desire to become a nurse took an unexpected turn when he had to choose between feelings of disgust and the needs of the patient. I am happy to say that Todd *did* become a nurse and has been working in some busy EDs—and he takes good care of his patients no matter how they smell. Erin, from chapter 3, never succeeded in introducing acupuncture to his ED. With the never-ending competition for resources, management never gave serious consideration to the idea. By denying Erin's request, the nursing managers were making what I saw to be a wise decision to set limits on what nurses are expected to know and do. By contrast, Sherry (from chapter 3) succeeded in the ED because she could see what needed to happen when time was of the essence.

We need to rethink the nursing scope of practice. The system we've adopted, with all its problems of litigation, regulation, and government control, has established a vague scope of practice that stifles creativity and offers little chance for growth. Nurses are warned to stay within the scope. But that prevents us from increasing our range of skills. Dr. Dan Tennenhouse, who teaches medical law at UCSF, told me that the scope of practice is actually whatever nurses typically do, which means if we're not already doing it, then by definition it is outside our scope. Changing this legal regime is one of the best ways for us to move the profession forward.

Nurses are human. We sometimes make mistakes, and that remains a challenge. The actual number of errors we make is assuredly far greater than is ever recorded. But because the "acceptable level of performance" has been idealized rather than being based on what is real, many nurses feel forced to hide mistakes, surround themselves with confidants, and bully those they may not trusted out of their workplaces. The *Just Culture* model seeks to recognize this problem and differentiate between errors made by nurses in the course of regular "safe" work and those that result from recklessness. But the model cannot work and make a difference without solid backing; instead, though, some managements treat the *Just Culture* model as a tool they can apply at their discretion, not as an overarching and *system* way of working. Sarah's honest mistakes (see chapter 4) put her under the microscope, where the *Just Culture* would call her reckless even as other nurses were behaving far more recklessly.

Bullying is a symptom of stress and excessive job demands. Nurses don't simply bully out of panic, but as a calculated way to protect themselves. It's is a form of risk management. We won't get rid of bullying without addressing excessive expectations. Then we can build solidarity as a group and as a profession and use *that* to achieve the same goals nurses falsely think can be achieved with bullying. Unions are a path to some of that solidarity, but becoming unionized is not going to solve all the problems that persist even where nurses are in unions.

Gina (chapter 5) faced this situation, but in her case the bullying was coming from certified nursing assistants, managers, and the hospital. The motivations of those working around her were not clear, but the result was the same. Her coworkers were powerless to help because they were under the same pressure to protect their jobs. Cynthia represents the well-meaning but naïve manager. Our hospitals are filled with nurses in leadership positions who are under some of the same pressures as the nurses on the floor. We can work together instead of against each other.

A Framework for Change

As this book notes, there are as many opportunities for improvement as there are problems encountered by nurses and the nursing profession. The future of nursing will be determined first and foremost by us, the nurses, and we must be the ones who take the needed steps. It's time for nurses to take control of our profession rather than waiting for others to fix the expectations and limits under which we work. The people who actually *work* in a profession know it best and should be the ones to establish policy. RNs outnumber all other categories healthcare providers, and there can be tremendous strength in numbers.

Six overarching recommendations tie together the many issues I've raised and provide a framework for moving forward.

1. Nurses need to be the ones to set appropriate limits. The single most important message in this book is that just as nurses are taking on more and more responsibility, they are doing so without the authority and control necessary to make their expanded roles workable. Of course, it's reasonable to expect a nurse to know her job duties, not make mistakes, and so on. However, the sum of these expectations is not reasonable and not doable. There was never any plan to set up the job description, so it should come as no surprise that these disparate elements are disjointed and often incompatible. Now that we have seen some of the results, and now that nursing has been professionalized for over a generation, we can recognize the effects of this lack of planning.

The starting point for defining the nurse's role is to adopt this perspective: What can an *individual* nurse reasonably accomplish safely and effectively? The answer requires looking at the process and making some difficult decisions. Any one person—even trained well for a profession—has a finite amount of attention, skills, resources, and abilities. Ask that person to do something that exceeds those limits, and it stands to reason that you ought to indicate what other expectations can be reduced. That, though, is not how it works in nursing: we're asked to work harder, multi-task, and when the job gets to be too much, we're expected not to reduce efforts in any area, and not to take any short cuts, but rather to reach out to our co-workers or get help from management. That is not sustainable.

Documentation and medication errors are especially prone to the problems of not setting appropriate limits. While the experts are advising us to chart only what is necessary and emphasize quality over quantity, the hospitals and our managers are telling us the opposite. Technology, in this respect, may do as much harm as good: while it makes recordkeeping easier, it has led us down a path where documentation is more important than patient care. As for medication errors, monitoring the 99 percent of them that do not affect patient safety is preventing us from focusing on the treatments that do matter. All the emphasis on that which can be measured and documented is crowding out the aspects of patient care that cannot. No wonder so many nurses turn to bullying to control the risk of being accused of errors we all make.

An overarching solution to limits and expectations is to reconsider the nurse's scope of practice. Today, we work under a scope of practice that is incomprehensible and provides little practical guidance. We should be looking for ways to expand our professional practice safely and prudently. The legal battles over professional boundaries make it clear there is a turf war going on. Instead of avoiding the conflict, we should simply acknowledge it and move forward with our goals.

2. Nurses must unionize—but a union won't solve every problem. Given the pressures and unrealistic expectations nurses face, it's little wonder that shortcuts have become standard practice and disciplinary actions against nurses are sporadic and often retaliatory. There is simply no way a nurse can fulfill the expectations made of her, protect her patient, and protect her job. A strong labor union is, therefore, absolutely necessary to give nurses the chance to do our jobs properly and keep those jobs. Without a labor union, a nurse can lose her job and her license in a moment—and with little recourse. Moving forward, a unionized workforce will bring stability that will help patients, hospitals, and nurses.

The nursing profession has this odd split between management and labor. Nurses are supposed to be professionals and leaders, but we are still workers and not management. As with people in many non-industrial jobs, we have bought into the notion that we are better than mere "laborers" and thus unions are not needed. Union rules and management practice have created a sharp division between the nurse and the manager. We call ourselves the nursing profession as if we are all working toward a common goal, yet we divide ourselves up into "labor" and "management."[1] That is why the need for nurses to unionize has not been more apparent.

For a nursing union to be strong, it needs to embrace long-term viability. Hospitals and a nurses union would both benefit from a long-term perspective. We have plenty of examples of cooperative labor-management systems in which nurses get paid well, the hospital gets the most talented workers, and management and the labor force are allies on a team. That should be a union's objective: not to be seen as an enemy of management, but to achieve a balance of forces.

That requires some give and take that may be unique to nursing jobs. Nurses should support nursing leaders instead of denying them moral legitimacy when hard decisions need to be made. For example, nurse managers need to discipline nurses, balance budgets, and distribute precious resources. The decision-making process of an individual nurse regarding the care of one patient is fundamentally different from a nurse manager deciding on matters related to healthcare outcomes on a wider scale.

Unfortunately, many nurses take management positions and leave their profession behind. I often wonder when nursing leaders in the hospitals I've worked at last took care of a patient. One way to address this is to ensure that nurses from all levels of the organization are actively engaged in decision making. Nurses who hold patient lives in their hands on a daily basis must not be subjected to rules and systems designed by others who may be out of touch with the demands of this profession. It is up to the bedside nurse to take initiatives and not wait for managers to ask for their opinions. Having a union is what ensures that the bedside nurse has a voice.

Even if all nurses are unionized, though, we need to be realistic that it is not a panacea for all the problems nurses face. Bullying, for instance, happens even in those work places that are unionized. Clearly, union protection is not a total solution, but it is the necessary start.

3. We must end the artificial "diagnosis" divide between nurses and doctors. Nurses have been taught to stay within the scope of nursing and even to fear that which is beyond that scope. "Leave it to the *real* experts," we're told. "Leave it to the doctors." This is nowhere more obvious than when it comes to the legal ability to make diagnoses. We work under a scope of practice that is incomprehensible and that does not provide much practical guidance. I see no reason why nurses need a scope of practice, as currently defined, when doctors work perfectly well with a medical scope of practice that is essentially open. Rather than shy away from these limits like something to be feared, we should be looking for ways to expand our professional practice safely and prudently. The legal battles over professional boundaries make it clear there is a turf war going on. Instead of avoiding the conflict, we should simply acknowledge it and move forward with our goals.

The dysfunctional system of nursing diagnoses, such as NANDA diagnoses, is a main hindrance to moving forward with the authority to diagnose.[2] The fact that there are multiple systems is bad enough. It makes a nurse look silly when she "diagnoses" a person with "readiness for enhanced spirituality" or any of the other bad choices. The solution is obvious: use medical diagnoses. Nurse practitioners are using them without any apologies to the nursing profession or to doctors. Nurses using medical diagnoses would not be a "betrayal" of our profession.

4. Nurses must be at the table when efficiency and productivity are discussed. Healthcare in this country is expensive. We pay far more per capita for healthcare than anywhere else in the developed world, but our outcomes do not come close to what should be reasonably expected. Nurses are a major expense in the healthcare system. As society struggles to find solutions to the cost problem, one thing is clear: given our importance in a person's overall healthcare, nurses are central to the discussion.

Productivity improvements cannot be achieved simply by making nurses work harder; we're already overloaded. The starting point must be to set appropriate limits on what a nurse can do, and have nurses be part of the process as hospitals make decisions about productivity. There will be financial consequences, which the nursing professional will need to address.

The corollary to productivity is efficiency—which is largely about getting more for less. This is a discussion nurses don't like; nurses have a tendency to have unrealistic expectations about money. Hospitals and other organizations have limits on what they can do based on their financial resources. They only operate because someone is paying the bills. Nurses, though, want to spend more time "caring" but typically don't care about who might be willing to pay for that. Meanwhile, nursing leaders that should appreciate the need for financial and organizational viability want to avoid appearing cold hearted.

As we look at the job demands put on us, we must also consider the resources needed to meet our expectations as well as those of our employers, especially the hospitals. We all want a nurse that takes that extra little time for the personal touch. We also want safe care. A nurse would love to have that extra time, but also to be well paid. At some point, we need to talk seriously about what contributes most to our healthcare and what nurses can do most efficiently.

And that's why we must be at the table when productivity and efficiency are discussed.

5. There needs to be more research about nursing. Some professional disciplines have vast research programs; the same cannot be said of nursing. Perhaps no other knowledge-based discipline has as few trained researchers as nursing. Less than one in every 100 nurses has a doctorate, and very few of those PhDs were trained to do research; nursing PhDs tend to focus on management and leadership. The average age of a nursing PhD student is close to 50, so even those who might engage in active post-doctorate research are relatively late in their careers.

As if this were not concerning enough, the proportion of nurses with doctorates is *less* than the proportion of the general public, by a large margin. In the United States, 1.7 percent of the population has a doctorate,* yet nursing, which is supposed to be professional, has almost half that amount. The end result is that the three million nurses in this country, and many others worldwide, are operating beneath their potential.

One major reason for this lack of research flows in large part from the fact that our profession does not reward knowledge development. Direct patient care nurses in hospitals make higher wages than nursing professors or researchers. No wonder nursing schools struggle to attract enough of the most talented to teach the next generation of nurses.

Career paths do not accommodate an acute care nurse who wants to teach or do research; unlike many other professions, nursing does not have hybrid practice/research positions that allow someone still working at a primary job to take time to participate in teaching or research.

Increasing research is a path towards becoming more sophisticated about our profession, reducing those things that do not contribute to patient care, and increasing those activities that do improve our efficiency. Nurse researchers, particularly those individuals with an understanding of acute care, can help use manage our workloads.

6. Nurse associations should be leading our profession. At present, nursing boards run our profession serving as the government's regulators. They set direction and priorities. We need to establish a different model for how our profession is run—and put newly empowered nurse associations at the forefront. After all, they represent us. The boards do not.

Yes, there are lots of nurses' associations, national and local, based on specialties or workplace. I could join any one of a dozen associations that fit my work role. That divides us as a community and often leads to competition for resources. We need to address that dispersion, and our associations will need to make some changes. But beyond that, we need our professional associations to take the lead in several areas that are now the purview of the boards. Our associations could be the ones issuing licenses and setting safety standards. If this sounds surprising, remember that some other countries do let their professional associations perform this role.

Nursing boards should continue to supervise the safety of nurses and the nursing profession, supervise the quality of nursing education, and to serve as advocates for patients. They should maintain their authority to discipline nurses and nursing schools that do not meet safety standards. But any roles that can be played by the associations should be.

Today, nursing schools routinely bring their students to nursing board meetings because the boards are in charge. Imagine representatives of our associations instead visit nursing schools and bring students in as members and into the decision-making process from the beginning of their careers. That would be possible if associations were leading our profession.

In short, we need to be giving our time, energy, and legitimacy to our professional associations, instead of to the nursing boards. Our associations ought to step up and drive changes. Nursing associations should be telling nursing boards what *we* want, where *we* want our nursing profession to be heading, and how *we* think that ought to happen.

***

Our national, and global, healthcare systems are at a critical juncture. Technology can do amazing things, but it cannot replace the human touch. Nurses have risen in a remarkably short time from handmaidens doing manual labor to independent clinical professionals. Consider the issues raised in these pages not as problems, but as growing pains. We nurses have more power than we think, and more wisdom than we utilize. By harnessing both, we will not only improve our profession; we can save lives.

Chapter 8 References

[1] Corwin, "The Professional Employee."
[2] Herdman, "Nursing Diagnoses 2012–14."

Appendix
Nevada's Unprofessional Conduct Regulation for Nurses[*]

NAC 632.890 **Unprofessional conduct.**

The Board will consider the following acts, among others, by a licensee or holder of a certificate as unprofessional conduct:

1. Discriminating on the basis of race, religious creed, color, national origin, age, disability, ancestry, sexual orientation or sex in the rendering of nursing services.
2. Performing acts beyond the scope of the practice of nursing.
3. Assuming duties and responsibilities within the practice of nursing without adequate training.
4. Assuming duties and responsibilities within the practice of nursing if competency is not maintained or the standards of competence are not satisfied, or both.
5. Disclosing the contents of the examination for licensure or certification, or soliciting, accepting or compiling information regarding the contents of the examination before, during or after its administration.
6. Assigning or delegating functions, tasks or responsibilities of licensed

or certified persons to unqualified persons.

7. Failing to supervise a person to whom functions of nursing are delegated or assigned, if responsible for supervising that person.

8. Failing to safeguard a patient from the incompetent, abusive or illegal practice of any person.

9. Practicing nursing while, with or without good cause, his or her physical, mental or emotional condition impairs his or her ability to act in a manner consistent with established or customary nursing standards, or both.

10. Practicing nursing, if any amount of alcohol or a controlled substance or dangerous drug that is not legally prescribed is present in the body of the nurse, nursing assistant or medication aide - certified as determined by a test of the blood, saliva, breath, hair or urine of the nurse, nursing assistant or medication aide - certified given while the nurse, nursing assistant or medication aide - certified is on duty.

11. Having present in the body of the nurse, nursing assistant or medication aide - certified alcohol or a controlled substance or dangerous drug that is not legally prescribed during a test of the blood, saliva, breath, hair or urine of the nurse, nursing assistant or medication aide - certified given as a condition of employment.

12. Failing to respect and maintain a patient's right to privacy.

13. Violating a patient's confidentiality.

14. Performing or offering to perform the functions of a licensee or holder of a certificate by false representation or under a false or an assumed name.

15. Failing to report the gross negligence of a licensee or holder of a certificate in the performance of his or her duties or a violation of the provisions of this chapter or chapter 632 of NRS.

16. Failing to document properly the administration of a controlled substance, including, but not limited to:

   (a) Failing to document the administration of a controlled substance on the Controlled Substance Administration Record, the patient's Medication Administration Record and the Nursing Progress Notes, including the patient's response to the medication;

   (b) Documenting as wastage a controlled substance and taking that controlled substance for personal or other use;

   (c) Failing to document the wastage of a controlled substance that was not legally administered to a patient;

(d) Soliciting the signature on any record of a person as a witness to the wastage of a controlled substance when that person did not witness the wastage; or

(e) Signing any record as a witness attesting to the wastage of a controlled substance which he or she did not actually witness.

17. Soliciting services or soliciting or borrowing money, materials or other property, or any combination thereof, from a:

(a) Patient;

(b) Family member of a patient;

(c) Person with significant personal ties to a patient, whether or not related by blood; or

(d) Legal representative of a patient.

18. Diverting supplies, equipment or drugs for personal or unauthorized use.

19. Aiding, abetting or assisting any person in performing any acts prohibited by law.

20. Inaccurate recording, falsifying or otherwise altering or destroying records.

21. Obtaining, possessing, furnishing or administering prescription drugs to any person, including himself or herself, except as directed by a person authorized by law to prescribe drugs.

22. Leaving an assignment without properly notifying the appropriate personnel or abandoning a patient in need of care.

23. Exploiting a patient for financial gain or offering, giving, soliciting or receiving fees or gifts for the referral of a:

(a) Patient;

(b) Family member of a patient;

(c) Person with significant personal ties to a patient, whether or not related by blood; or

(d) Legal representative of a patient.

24. Failing to collaborate with other members of a health care team as necessary to meet the health needs of a patient.

25. Failing to observe the conditions, signs and symptoms of a patient, to record the information or to report significant changes to the appropriate persons.

26. Failing to abide by any state or federal statute or regulation relating to the practice of nursing.

27. Failing to perform nursing functions in a manner consistent with

established or customary standards.

28. Causing a patient or the family of the patient physical, mental or emotional harm by taking direct or indirect actions or failing to take appropriate actions.

29. Engaging in sexual contact with a patient or client.

30. Failing as a chief nurse to:

(a) Institute standards of nursing practice so that safe and effective nursing care is provided to patients;

(b) Institute standards of competent organizational management and management of human resources so that safe and effective nursing care is provided to patients; or

(c) Create a safe and effective environment, including the failure to assess the knowledge, skills and ability of a licensee or holder of a certificate and determine his or her competence to carry out the requirements of his or her job.

31. Failing to report the unauthorized practice of nursing.

32. Endangering the safety of the general public, patients, clients or coworkers by making actual or implied threats of violence or carrying out an act of violence.

33. Abusing a patient.

34. Neglecting a patient.

35. Misappropriating the property of a patient.

36. Failing to comply with a condition, limitation or restriction which has been placed on his or her license or certificate.

37. Engaging in the practice of nursing or performing the services of a nursing assistant or medication aide - certified without a license or certificate issued pursuant to the provisions of this chapter and chapter 632 of NRS.

38. Displaying a license, certificate, diploma or permit, or a copy of a license, certificate, diploma or permit, which has been fraudulently purchased, issued, counterfeited or materially altered.

39. Engaging in a pattern of conduct that demonstrates failure to exercise the knowledge, skills, and abilities using the methods ordinarily exercised by a reasonable and prudent nurse to protect the public.

40. Committing an error in the administration or delivery of medication to a patient.

41. Failing to cooperate with an investigation conducted by the Board.

42. Engaging in any other unprofessional conduct with a patient or client

that the Board determines is outside the professional boundaries generally considered acceptable in the profession, including, without limitation, a violation of the guidelines of the American Nurses Association or the National Council of State Boards of Nursing concerning the appropriate use of social media.

(Added to NAC by Bd. of Nursing, eff. 8-5-86; A 6-30-88; 2-6-90; 11-19-93; 5-18-94; 5-9-96; R029-97, 1-26-98; R081-06, 6-28-2006; R196-07, 4-17-2008; R063-08, 9-18-2008; R112-11, 2-15-2012)

Appendix References
* https://www.leg.state.nv.us/NAC/NAC-632.html#NAC632Sec890. "NRS" is a reference to the Nevada Revised Statutes.

Bibliography

Abramson, Norman S, Karen Silvasy Wald, Ake NA Grenvik, Deborah Robinson, and James V. Snyder. "Adverse Occurrences in Intensive Care Units." *Journal of the American Medical Association* 244, no. 14 (1980): 1582–1584.

Achen, Christopher H., and Larry M. Bartels, *Democracy for Realists: Why Elections Do Not Produce Responsive Governments* (Princeton, NJ: Princeton University Press, 2016).

AFL-CIO, "Nursing: A Profile of the Profession." Fact Sheet, 2013. https://dpeaflcio.org/wp-content/uploads/nursing-2013.pdf

Aiken, Linda H., Sean P. Clarke, Robyn B. Cheung, Douglas M. Sloane, and Jeffrey H. Silber. "Educational Levels of Hospital Nurses and Surgical Patient Mortality." *Journal of the American Medical Association* 290, no. 12 (2003): 1617–1623.

_____, Sean P. Clarke, Douglas M. Sloane, Julie A. Sochalski, Reinhard Busse, Heather Clarke, Phyllis Giovannetti, Jennifer Hunt, Anne Marie Rafferty, and Judith Shamian. "Nurses' Report on Hospital Care in Five Countries." *Health Affairs* 20, no. 3 (2001): pp. 43–53.

_____, Sean P. Clarke, Douglas M. Sloane, Julie Sochalski, and Jeffrey H. Silber. "Hospital Nurse Staffing and Patient Mortality, Nurse Burnout, and Job Satisfaction." *Journal of the American Medical Association* 288, no. 16 (2002): 1987–1993.

_____, Douglas M. Sloane, Luk Bruyneel, Luk., Koen Van den Heede, Koen, Walter Sermeus, and Rn4cast Consortium. "Nurses' Reports of Working Conditions and Hospital Quality of Care in 12 Countries in Europe." *International Journal of Nursing Studies* 50, no. 2 (2013): 143–153.

_____, Douglas M. Sloane, Jeannie P. Cimiotti, Sean P. Clarke, Linda Flynn, Jean Ann Seago, Joanne Spetz, and Herbert L. Smith. "Implications of the California Nurse Staffing Mandate for Other States." *Health Services Research*

45, no. 4 (2010): 904–921.

Allan, Elizabeth L., and Kenneth N. Barker. "Fundamentals of Medication Error Research. *American Journal of Hospital Pharmacy* 47, no 3 (1990): 555–571.

American Society of Hospital Pharmacists (AHSP). "ASHP Guidelines on Preventing Medication Errors in Hospitals. *American Journal of Hospital Pharmacists* 50 (1993): 305–314.

Ammenwerth, Elske, Petra Schnell-Inderst, Christof Machan, and Uwe Siebert. "The Effect of Electronic Prescribing on Medication Errors and Adverse Drug Events: A Systematic Review." *Journal of the American Medical Informatics Association* 15, no. 5 (2008): 585–600.

Antonow, Juli A., Anne B. Smith, and Michael P. Silver. "Medication Error Reporting: A Survey of Nursing Staff." *Journal of Nursing Care Quality* 15, no. 1 (2000): 42–48.

Audit Commission, *A Spoonful of Sugar: Medicines Management in NHS Hospitals* (London: Audit Commission, 2001).

Baker, Helen M. "Rules Outside the Rules for Administration of Medication: A Study in New South Wales, Australia." *Image: The Journal of Nursing Scholarship* 29, no. 22 (1997): 155–158.

Barker, Kenneth N., Elizabeth A. Flynn, Ginette A. Pepper, David W. Bates, and Robert L. Mikeal, Robert L. "Medication Errors Observed in 36 Health Care Facilities." *Archives of Internal Medicine* 162, no. 16 (2002): 1897–1903.

Benner, Patricia, *From Novice to Expert: Excellence and Power in Clinical Nursing Practice, Commemorative Edition* (Upper Saddle River, NJ: Prentice Hall, 2001).

Bickel, Janet. "Why Do Women Hamper Other Women?" *Journal of Women's Health* 23, no. 5 (2014): 365–367.

Bilgel, Nazan, Serpil Aytaç, and Nuran Bayram. "Bullying in Turkish White-Collar Workers." *Occupational Medicine* 56, no. 4 (2006): 226–231.

Board of Registered Nursing, State of California. "An Explanation of the Scope of RN Practice Including Standardized Procedures." Rev. 07/1997, 01/2011. https://www.rn.ca.gov/pdfs/regulations/npr-b-03.pdf

Bradley, Elizabeth, Jeph Herrin, Yongfei Wang, Barbara A. Barton, Tashonna R. Webster, Jennifer A. Mattera, Sarah A. Roumanis, *et al.* "Strategies for Reducing the Door-to-Balloon Time in Acute Myocardial Infarction." *New England Journal of Medicine* 355, no. 22 (2006): 2308–2320.

Bradshaw, Ann. "Measuring Nursing Care and Compassion: The McDonaldised Nurse?" *Journal of Medical Ethics* 35, no. 8 (2009): 465–468.

———, *The Project 2000 Nurse: The Remaking of British General Nursing, 1978–2000* (New York: Wiley, 2001).

Brady, Anne-Marie, Anne-Marie Malone, and Sandra Fleming. "A Literature Review of the Individual and Systems Factors that Contribute to Medication Errors in Nursing Practice." *Journal of Nursing Management* 17, no. 6 (2009): 679–697.

Brennan, Troyen A., Lucian L. Leape, Nan M. Laird, Liesi Hebert, Russell Localio, Ann G. Lawthers, Joseph P. Newhouse, Paul C. Weiler, and Howard H. Hiatt. "Incidence of Adverse Events and Negligence in Jospitalized Patients: Results of the Harvard Medical Practice Study I. *New England Journal of Medicine* 324, no. 6 (1991): 370–376.

Brown, Theresa, *The Shift: One Nurse, Twelve Hours, Four Patients' Lives* (Chapel Hill, NC: Algonquin Books, 2015).

Burgess, Lorraine, Fiona Irvine, and Akhtar Wallymahmed. "Personality, Stress and Coping in Intensive Care Nurses: A Descriptive Exploratory Study." *Nursing in Critical Care* 15, no. 3 (2010): 129–140.

Choy, Catherine C., *Empire of Care: Nursing and Migration in Filipino American History* (Durham, NC: Duke University Press, 2003).

Corwin, Ronald G., "The Professional Employee: A Study of Conflict in Nursing Roles." *American Journal of Sociology* 66, no. 6: 604–615.

Cosby, Karen S., and Pat Croskerry. "Profiles in Patient Safety: Authority Gradients in Medical Error." *Academy of Emergency Medicine* 11, no. 12 (2004): 1341–1345.

Curtis, Janette, Isla Bowen, and Amanda Reid. "You Have No Credibility: Nursing Students' Experiences of Horizontal Violence." *Nurse Education in Practice* 7, no. 3 (2007): 156–163.

Danish Nursing Organization, "Solidaritetsarbejde." https://dsr.dk/om-dsr/

———, "Welcome to DNO." https://dsr.dk/om-dsr/kontakt-dsr/welcome-to-dno

D'Ambra, Amanda M., and Diane R. Andrews. "Incivility, Retention and New Graduate Nurses: An Integrated Review of the Literature." *Journal of Nursing Management* 22, no. 6 (2014): 735–742.

Donelan, Karen, Peter Buerhaus, Catherine DesRoches, Robert Dittus, and David Dutwin. "Public Perceptions of Nursing Careers: The Influence of the Media and Nursing Shortages." *Nursing Economics* 26, no. 3 (2008): 143–165.

European Federation of Nurses Associations, "History." http://www.efnweb.be/?page_id=766

Freire, Paulo, *Pedagogy of the Oppresses* (New York: Seabury, 1973).

Garlo, Dolores M. "Critical Care Nurses: A Case for Legal Recognition of the Growing Responsibilities and Accountability in the Nursing Profession." *Journal of Contemporary Law* 11 (1984): 239.

Gawande, Atul, *The Checklist Manifesto: How to Get Things Right* (New York: Picador, 2011).

Gladstone, Jill. "Drug Administration Errors: A Study into the Factors Underlying the Occurrence and Reporting of Drug Errors in a District

General Hospital." *Journal of Advanced Nursing* 22, no. 4 (1995): 628–637.

Good, Vicki. "Giving thanks … for failure." *Bold Voices*. American Association of Critical Care Nurses. November 2013: 22.

Gordon, Suzanne, and Siobhan Nelson. "An End to Angels." *AJN The American Journal of Nursing* 105, no. 5 (2005): 62–69.

Gorrell, Gena K. *Heart and Soul: The Story of Florence Nightingale* (Toronto: Tundra Books, 2000).

Graeber, Charles. *The Good Nurse: A True Story of Medicine, Madnes, and Murder* (New York: Twelve, 2013).

Guido, Ginny W., *Legal and Ethical Issues in Nursing*, 5th ed. (New York: Pearson, 2010).

Health Resources and Services Administration (HRSA), U.S. Department of Health and Human Services. "The Registered Nurse Population: Findings from the 2008 National Sample Survey of Registered Nurses." September 2010. Washington, DC: bhw.hrsa.gov/sites/default/files/bhw/nchwa/rnsurveyfinal.pdf

Herdman, T.H., *Nursing Diagnoses 2012–14: Definitions and Classification.* (New York: John Wiley & Sons, 2012).

Hill, D.S., & Crow, "Vietnam Nurse Project: Teaching in Hanoi. *Nursing2019* 43, no. 2 (2013): 55–59.

Hochschild, Arlie, *The Managed Heart: Commercialization of Human Feeling* (Berkeley, CA: University of California Press, 1983).

Hutchinson, Marie, Margaret Vickers, Debra Jackson, and Lesley Wilkes. "Workplace Bullying in Nursing: Towards a More Critical Organizational Perspective." *Nursing Inquiry* 13, no. 2 (2006): 118–126.

International Labour Organization, "About the ILO," https://www.ilo.org/global/about-the-ilo/lang--en/index.htm

Jack, Dana Crowley, *Behind the Mask: Destruction and Creativity in Women's Aggression* (Cambridge, MA: Harvard University Press, 1999).

———, *Silencing the Self: Women and Depression* (Cambridge, MA: Harvard University Press, 1991).

Jameton, Andrew, *Nursing Practice: The Ethical Issues* (Englewood Cliffs, NJ: Prentice-Hall, 1984).

Johnson, Martin. "Drugs and Discipline." *Senior Nurse* 6, no. 2 (1987): 14–16.

Kahneman, Daniel, *Thinking, Fast and Slow* (New York: Farrar, Straus, and Giroux, 2013).

———, Paul Slovic, and Amos Tversky, eds., *Judgment Under Uncertainty: Heuristics and Biases* (New York: Cambridge University Press, 1987).

——— and Amos Tversky, eds., *Choices, Values, and Frames* (New York: Cambridge University Press, 2000).

Karleson, Kristine A., Thomas J. Hendrix, and Maureen O'Malley. "Medical Error Reporting in America: A Changing Landscape." *Quality Management in*

Health Care 18, no. 1 (2009): 59–70.

Keers, Richard N., Steven D. Williams, Jonathan Cooke, and Darren M. Ashcroft. "Causes of Medical Administration Errors in Hospitals: A Systematic Review of Quantitative and Qualitative Evidence. *Drug Safety* 36, no. 11 (2013): 1047–1067.

Keers, Richard N., Steven D. Williams, Jonathan Cooke, Tanya Walsh, and Darren M. Ashcroft. "Impact of Interventions Designed to Reduce Medication Administration Errors in Hospitals: A Systematic review. *Drug Safety* 37, no. 5 (2014): 317–332.

Kingma, Mireille, *Nurses on the Move: Migration and the Global Health Care Economy* (Ithaca, NY: ILR Press, 2005).

Kochan, Thomas A., Adrienne E. Eaton, Robert B. McKersie, and Paul S. Adler, *Healing Together: The Labor-Management Partnership at Kaiser Permanente* (Ithaca, NY: ILR Press, 2009).

Kyle, Tanya. "The Concept of Caring: A Review of the Literature." *Journal of Advanced Nursing* 21, no. 3 (1995): 506–514.

Larson, Patricia. "Important Nurse Caring Behaviors Perceived by Patients with Cancer." *Oncology Nursing Forum* 11 (1984): 46–50.

Leape, Lucian L. "Apology for Errors: Whose Responsibility? *Frontiers of Health Services Management* 28, no. 3 (2012): 3–12.

Leape, Lucian L. "Scope of Problem and History of Patient Safety." *Obstetrics and Gynecology Clinics of North America* 35, no. 1 (2008): 1–10.

Leape, Lucian L., and Donald M. Berwick. "Five years after To Err is Human." *Journal of the American Medical Association* 293, 19 (2005): 2378.

Li, Y.I.N., and Cheryl B. Jones. "A Literature Review of Nursing Turnover Costs." *Journal of Nursing Management* 21, no. 3 (2013): 405–418.

Makary, Matin A., and Michael Daniel. "Medical Error—The Third Leading Cause of Death in the US. *British Medical Journal* 353 (2016): i2139.

Manias, Elizabeth. "Detection of Medication-Related Problems in Hospital Practice: A Review." *British Journal of Clinical Pharmacology* 76, no. 1 (2013): 7–20.

Manthous, Constantine A. "Labor Unions in Medicine: The Intersection of Patient Advocacy and Self-advocacy. *Medical Care* 52, no. 5 (2014): 387–392.

Marx, David. "Patient Safety and the 'Just Culture': A Primer for Health Care Executives." Columbia University, April 17, 2001.

Mealer, Meredith L, April Shelton, Britt Berg, Barbara Rothbaum, and Marc Moss. "Increased Prevalence of Post-Traumatic Stress Disorder Symptoms in Critical Care Nurses." *American Journal of Respiratory and Critical Care Medicine* 175, no. 7 (2007): 693–697.

Menzies, Isabel E.P. "A Case-Study in the Functioning of Social Systems as a Defense Against Anxiety: A Report on a Study of the Nursing Service of a General Hospital." *Human Relations* 13, no. 2 (1960): 95–121.

National Center for Health Workforce Analysis. *The Future of the Nursing Workforce: National- and State-Level Projections, 2012–2025* (Rockville, MD: National Center for Health Workforce Analysis, 2014).

National Council of State Boards of Nursing. "2013 Canadian RN Practice Analysis: Applicability of the 2013 NCLEX-RN® Test Plan to the Canadian Testing Population. Research Brief, Vol. 60 (May 2014.) www.ncsbn.org/14_Canadian_Practice_Analysis_vol60.pdf

———, "NCSBN Award Ceremony to Honor Outstanding Nurse Regulators," June 13, 2017, https://www.ncsbn.org/10744.htm.

———, "Nurse Licensure Compact," https://www.ncsbn.org/nurse-licensure-compact.htm .

Neal-Boylan, Leslie, *The Nurse's Reality Shift: Using History to Transform the Future* (Indianapolis: Sigma Theta Tau International, 2014).

Norton, Michael I., Jeana H. Frost, and Dan Ariely. "Less Is Often More, but Not Always: Additional Evidence that Familiarity Breeds Contempt and a Call for Future *Research. Journal of Personality and Social Psychology* 105, no. 6 (2013): 921–923.

Nurse.org, "Highest Paying States for Registered Nurses," April 9, 2018, https://nurse.org/articles/highest-paying-states-for-registered-nurses/.

Phillips, Pauline. A Deconstruction of Caring. *Journal of Advanced Nursing* 18, no. 10 (1993): 1554–1558.

Record Research Staff. "Anderson man arrested after threatening to shoot himself and others in Mercy's emergency room." *Redding Record,* January 15, 2011.

Rhodes, Marilyn K., Arlene H. Morris, and Ramonda B. Lazenby. "Nursing at Its Best: Competent and Caring." *OJIN: The Online Journal of Issues in Nursing* 16, no. 2 (2011): 10.

Roberts, Susan Jo. "Oppressed Group Behavior: Implications for Nursing. *Advances in Nursing Science* 5, no. 4 (1983): 21–30.

Robertson, Kathy. "Nurses (still) wanted." *Sacramento Business Journal,* January 13, 2008.

Rosenberg, Charles E., *Our Present Complaint: American Medicine, Then and Now* (Baltimore, MD: John Hopkins University Press, 2007).

Royal College of Surgeons in Ireland, "About RCSI Bahrain." https://www.rcsi.com/bahrain/about-rcsi-bahrain

Schmidt, Eric, and Jonathan Rosenberg, *How Google Works* (New York: Grand Central Publishing, 2014).

Scott, Anthony, Julia Witt, Christine Duffield, and Guyonne Kalb. "What Do Nurses and Midwives Value About their Jobs? Results from a Discrete Choice Experiment." *Journal of Health Services Research & Policy* 20, no. 1 (2015)31–38.

Semega, Jessica. "Median Household Income for States: 2007 and 2008

American Community Surveys." U.S. Census Bureau (2009).

Smith, Barbara Peters. "Florida Is Facing Another Nursing Shortage." *Sarasota (Florida) Herald-Tribune*, March 16, 2012.

Smith, Marlaine C., Marian C. Turkel, and Zane Robinson Wolf, *Caring in Nursing Classics* (New York: Springer, 2012).

Smith, Pam, *The Emotional Labour of Nursing: How Nurses Care* (London: Palgrave, 1992).

Sochalski, Julie. (2002). Nursing Shortage Redux: Turning the Corner on an Enduring Problem. *Health Affairs* 21, no. 5 (2002): 157–164.

Spetz, Joanne, and Carolina Herrera, Carolina. "Changes in Nurse Satisfaction in California, 2004 to 2008." *Journal of Nursing Management* 18, no. 5 (2010): 564–572.

Strickland, Ora Lea. "Foreword." In Jean Watson, ed., *Assessing and Measuring Caring in Nursing and Health Sciences* (New York: Springer, 2008), xiii.

Suresh, Gautham, Jeffrey D. Horbar, Paul Plsek, James Gray, William H. Edwards, Patricia H. Shiono, Robert Ursprung, Julianne Nickerson, Jerold F. Lucey, and Donald Goldmann. "Voluntary Anonymous Reporting of Medical Errors for Neonatal Intensive Care." *Pediatrics* 113, no. 6 (2004): 1609–1618.

Sweller, John. "Cognitive Load During Problem Solving: Effects on Learning." *Cognitive Science* 12, no. 2 (1988): 257–285.

Taxis, Katja., and Nicholas Barber "Causes of Intravenous Medication Errors: An Ethnographic Study." *BMJ Quality & Safety* 12, no. 5 (2003): 343–347.

Tennant, Christopher, Pauline Langeluddecke, and Don Byrne. "The Concept of Stress. *Australia & New Zealand Journal of Psychiatry* 19, no. 2 (1985): 113–118.

Thomas, Sandra P. *Transforming Nurses' Anger and Pain: Steps Toward Healing* (New York: Springer, 1998).

Topol, Eric, *The Patient Will See You Now: The Future of Medicine Is In Your Hands* (New York: Basic Books, 2015).

Vessey, Judith A., Rosanna F. DeMarco, and Rachel DiFazio. "Bullying, Harassment, and Horizontal Violence in the Nursing Workforce." In Annette Debisette and Judith Vessey, eds., *Annual Review of Nursing Research* Vol. 28, chap. 6 (New York: Springer, 2011).

———, Rosanna F. DeMarco, Donna A. Gaffney, and Wendy C. Budin. "Bullying of Staff Registered Nurses in the Workplace: A Preliminary Study for Developing Personal and Organizational Strategies for the Transformation of Hostile to Health Workplace Environments." *Journal of Professional Nursing* 25, no. 5 (200): 299–306.

Watson, Jean, ed., *Assessing and Measuring Caring in Nursing and Health Sciences* (New York: Springer, 2008).

———, *Human Caring Science: A Theory of Nursing* (Burlington, MA: Jones &

Bartlett Learning, 2011).

Watson, Roger. "Clinical Competence: Starship Enterprise or Straitjacket?" *Nurse Education Today* 22, no. 6 (2002): 476–480.

Weinberg, Dana Beth, *Code Creen: Money-Driven Hospitals and the Dismantling of Nursing* (Ithaca, NY: ILR Press, 2003).

Weingarten, Gene. "Fatal distraction: Forgetting a child in the backseat of a car is a horrifying mistake. Is it a crime?" *Washington Post*, March 8, 2009

Williams, Angela. "A Literature Review on the Concept of Intimacy in Nursing." *Journal of Advanced Nursing* 33, no. 5 (2001): 660–667.

Wolf, Zane Robinson, Eileen Riviello Giardino, Patricia A. Osborne, and Marguerite Stahley. "Dimensions of Nurse Caring." *Image: The Journal of Nursing Scholarship* 26, no. 2 (1994): 107–112.

Zalumas, Jacqueline, *Caring in Crisis: An Oral History of Critical Care Nursing* (Philadelphia, PA: University of Pennsylvania Press, 1995).

Index

Brady, Anne-Marie, 98

Brown, Theresa, 115

Brown v. Board of Education, 137, 149

bullying, 4, 31, 70, 103–105; by "caring" nurse, 54; causes of, 112–117, 134, 203, 204; gender issues with, 111–112; incidence of, 111; *Just Culture* and, 198; no-tolerance policy of, 113; by reporting errors, 8, 15–17, 87–88, 101, 201; as risk management, 110–117; unions and, 203, 206

Burhans, Linda, 97

burnout, 7, 56, 108, 119. *See also* overwork

California Board of Registered Nurses, 16–19, 21, 148; NCLEX data and, 79; nurse-to-patient ratios and, 108; on scope of practice, 82–83

cardiopulmonary resuscitation (CPR): disciplinary actions from, 136, 148; injuries from, 74

caring, 8, 30, 34–36, 201; bullying and, 54; conflicts with, 39–53; definitions of, 34–36, 40, 51; doctors and, 52–53; gender issues with, 53–56; holistic, 53; instrumental, 40; professionalism and, 35, 39, 50, 56–58; quantification of, 51–52; tautology of, 51; Watson on, 35–36, 38–39, 50–51

Cattaneo, Umberto, 179

certified nursing assistants (CNAs), 80, 103–104, 111, 113, 203

Chamberlain College of Nursing (Nevada), 25–27

chaplain visits, 47

Codam, Majbritt, 168–169

Colorado Board of Nursing, 36–38, 141, 146–148

Columbine High School massacre (1999), 38–39

communication, 63, 110–111; gendered styles of, 53; with patients, 59; with patients' families, 61

community healthcare, 7

competency, 52, 69–71

Complaint Evaluation Tool, 97

Connecticut Board of Nursing, 125

continuing education, 129

Cooperation Council for the Arab States of the Gulf, 171

Corrective Action Decision Tree, 118

Cosby, Karen S., 101

Council for Graduates of Foreign Nursing Schools (CGFNS), 176

Crimean War (1853–1856), 33

critical thinking skills, 7, 62

Croskerry, Pat, 101

Crow, Greg, 163–164

Cullen, Charles, 42

Daniel, Michael, 89–90

Decent Work Across Borders (organization), 179

Delaware Board of Nursing, 148

Denmark, 167–171

doctors, 6–7, 44–45, 52–53; "caring" by, 52; chain of command of, 113; errors by, 89–90, 93, 100–101; nurses and, 6–7, 52–53, 104–105, 113, 199; salaries of, 44; scope of practice of, 80, 82, 84, 206

Dubai, 185–186. *See also* United Arab Emirates

East Timor, 163, 176

efficiency/productivity measures, 67–68, 206–207

electronic health records, 2, 15, 66, 94–95, 204. *See also* information systems

emergency medical technicians (EMTs), 11, 13, 15–18; training of, viii, 76–77

emotional intelligence, 74

emotional involvement, 57, 201; boundaries of, 49, 145–146

emotional labor, 40, 50

errors, 57, 68, 87–88; bullying by reporting, 8, 15–17, 87–88, 101, 201; checklists for avoiding, 75–76; control of, 95–102, 204; incidence of, 94–95; Institute of Medicine's report on, 91, 91; *Just Culture* approach to, 198–199; medication, 11–12, 88–102, 104–105, 197; nonreporting of, 67, 96–98; nurses accusing other nurses of, 1–2, 11–12, 39, 201; patient abuse and, 11–12; reportable, 64, 95–97, 96; responsibility for, 52, 200; scope of practice and, 80; types of, 92–93, 96; underreporting of, 96–97, 202; unprofessional conduct and, 51, 128–129, 211–215

ethical standards, 57–58

European Union, 169–170

existential-phenomenological-spiritual factors, 36

expatriate nurses, 15, 44, 119, 168, 171; accreditation of, 176; in Bahrain, 193; Decent Work Across Borders and, 179; qualifications of, 77; in United Arab Emirates, 187. *See also* global nursing

Forrest, Elena, 80–81

Freire, Paulo, 112

gaming the system, 4–5, 51–52; by breaking rules, 67; cliques and, 87, 115, 119, 201; medication errors and, 93–94; scope of practice and, 81

Garner, Janie, 121–122

Gawande, Atul, 64, 75

Gelenidze, Ia, 183–192

gender issues, 41; in Arab countries, 181–183; with bullying, 111–112; with caring, 53–56

Georgia, Republic of, 183

Gladstone, Jill, 94–95

global nursing, 44, 77, 142, 155–195, 209; in Africa, 156–157, 170, 175; Council for Graduates of Foreign Nursing Schools and, 176; in Denmark, 167–171; in Maldives, 160–161; in Middle East, 171–177, 180–194; in New Zealand, 157–160; in Poland, 165–166; in Sri Lanka, 161–163; in Vietnam, 163–165. *See also* expatriate nurses

Gomez, Mariela, 160–162, 174, 183–186, 190, 193

Google Corporation, 68

Gordon, Suzanne, 28, 33–34, 122

Gulf Cooperation Council (GCC), 171n
gun violence, 39

Harvard Medical Practice Study, 91
Hedges, Matthew, 185
heuristics, 74–75
Hippocratic oath, 33
HIV/AIDS, 156–157, 170
Hochschild, Arlie, 40, 50
holistic care, 53
home care nursing, 117
home healthcare, 7
homosexuality. *See* LGBTQ issues

in-service training, 79
incident reports, 11, 93, 114
India, 171, 174, 179, 187
Indonesia, 163, 176
information systems, 2, 15, 64–66, 104; chart reviews and, 93; improving of, 204;
      medication orders and, 66, 94–95
Institute of Medicine (IOM), 91, 100
International Council of Nurses (ICN), 158, 165, 172, 174–178, 182, 194–195
International Labour Organization (ILO), 172–174, 178–179
interview techniques, 69–70
intra-osseus needles, 72–73
Iowa Board of Nursing, 130–132
ITT Technical Institute, 23

job interviews, 69–70
job performance, 113; criteria of, 4, 8; tests of, 36–37, 78, 146
job responsibilities, 3–5, 56–57, 203–204. *See also* scope of practice
job satisfaction, 7, 43, 48–49
job security, 119
Johnson, Martin, 100
Joint Commission on Accreditation of Healthcare Organizations (JCAHO), 197–198
Jordan, 171–172
Just Culture, 8, 19–20, 25, 31, 71, 197; advantages of, 198; definitions of, 89, 97; job
      security and, 119; measures of, 63–64; on nursing errors, 202; unionization and,
      118

Kahneman, Daniel, 74
Kaiser Permanente, 30, 64, 122, 199
Kansas Board of Nursing, 149–152
Karleson, Kristine, 96
Kennedy, Annette, 182
Khashoggi, Jamal, 185

Phillips, Pauline, 51
physicians. *See* doctors
Poland, 165–166
Porche, Demetrius, 127, 129, 138–139
post-traumatic stress disorder (PTSD), 109
power gradients, 101–102, 119, 126–127
preceptors, 62–63, 77, 88, 198
prednisolone, 97–98
productivity/efficiency measures, 67–68, 206–207
professionalism, 199; caring and, 35, 39, 50, 56–58; definitions of, 56; emotional boundaries and, 49; emotional involvement and??, 57–58; nurses' biases and, 47–48; salaries and, 44–45; standards of, 51, 128–129, 211–215
Puckett, Theresa, 120–121

Qatar, 171n
quality improvement programs, 197, 206–207

racial issues, 41–42, 47–48, 104; in Arkansas, 135, 137; ethnicity and, 119
"red man" syndrome, 89
registered nurses (RNs), 6; demographics of, 3, 5, 29; unionization of, 103
registry nurses, 67–68, 94–95, 197, 200
regulatory agencies, 200
risk management, bullying as, 110–117
Roberts, Susan Jo, 112–113
Royal College of Surgeons in Ireland (RCSI), 193

Saffar, Rula al-, 185–186
salaries: of doctors, 44; of nurses, 3, 43–45, 143, 168, 169
Saudi Arabia, 171n, 175, 180–182, 185, 194
scope of practice: of doctors, 80, 82, 84, 206; of nurses, 3–7, 24, 79–85, 198, 202–204, 206
Show Me Your Stethoscope (organization), 121–122
"smarts," 201–202; definitions of, 8, 31, 62; EMTs with, 76
social media, 145
South Africa, 47, 156, 175
spiritual care, 36, 66
Sri Lanka, 161–163
Stievano, Alessandro, 175, 176
stress, 105–110, 201; acute versus chronic, 106; moral distress and, 108–109
Strickland, Ora Lea, 35
stroke code, 75
substance abuse, 108, 112, 133–135
Swaziland, 156–157, 170
Switzerland, 172–180, 184
Syria, 172

Made in the USA
San Bernardino, CA
16 February 2020

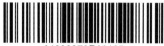